Independent and Supplementary Prescribing

An Essential Guide
Second edition

Independent and Supplementary Prescribing

An Essential Guide
Second edition

Edited by

Molly Courtenay
Matt Griffiths

Foreword by

June Crown CBE

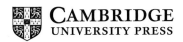

CAMBRIDGE
UNIVERSITY PRESS

CAMBRIDGE UNIVERSITY PRESS
Cambridge, New York, Melbourne, Madrid, Cape Town,
Singapore, São Paulo, Delhi, Tokyo, Mexico City

Cambridge University Press
The Edinburgh Building, Cambridge CB2 8RU, UK

Published in the United States of America by Cambridge University Press,
New York

www.cambridge.org
Information on this title: www.cambridge.org/9780521125208
© Cambridge University Press 2010

First edition published by Greenwich Medical Media 2004
This edition published by Cambridge University Press 2010

First published 2010
Reprinted 2011

Printed in the United Kingdom at the University Press, Cambridge

A catalogue record for this publication is available from the British Library

Library of Congress Cataloguing in Publication Data

Independent and supplementary prescribing : an essential guide / edited by
Molly Courtenay, Matt Griffiths; foreword by June Crown. – 2nd ed.
    p. ; cm.
Includes bibliographical references and index.
ISBN 978-0-521-12520-8 (pbk.)
1. Drugs–Prescribing. 2. Nurse practitioners–Prescription privileges.
I. Courtenay, Molly. II. Griffiths, Matt. III. Title.
[DNLM: 1. Drug Prescriptions. 2. Allied Health Personnel. 3. Drug
Therapy–methods. 4. Nurse's Role. 5. Pharmaceutical
Preparations–administration & dosage. 6. Pharmacists. QV 748 I38 2010]

RM138.I53 2010
615.1–dc22   2010009143

ISBN 978-0-521-12520-8 Paperback

Contents

Contributors

John Adams RGN, MA, MPhil
Senior Lecturer
Faculty of Health and Social Care
Peterborough District Hospital
Anglia Ruskin University
Peterborough, UK

Anne Baird RGN, MA
Nurse Practitioner and Associate
Lecturer
Porter Brook Medical Centre,
Sheffield and
Sheffield University and Sheffield
Hallam University
Sheffield, UK

**Polly Buchanan RGN, RM, ONC,
DipN, BSc (Hons)**
Department of Chemistry
King's College London
London, UK

Gillian Cavell
King's College Hospital
Denmark Hill
London, UK

**Stephen R. Chapman BSc (Hons), PhD,
Cert H Econ, FRSM, MRPharmS**
Professor of Prescribing Studies
Technical Development
School of Pharmacy
Keele University
Staffordshire, UK

**Michele Cossey MSc,
BPharm (Hons), MRPharmS**
Prescribing and Pharmacy Lead
NHS Yorkshire and the Humber
York, UK

**Molly Courtenay PhD, MSc, BSc,
CertEd, RGN, RNT**
Professor, Division of Health

and Social Care
University of Surrey
Marlow
Surrey, UK

Alison G. Eggleton MEd, MSc, BSc, SP
Principal Pharmacist, Education
and Training
Addenbrooke's Hospital
Cambridge, UK

**Mark Gagan RN, RNT, LLM, PGDip
Social Research, CertEd**
Senior Lecturer
Bournemouth University School of
Health and Social Care
Bournemouth, UK

**Trudy Granby RN, DN, MSc Clinical
Nursing**
Assistant Director, Prescribing and
Development Support
NPC Plus
Keele University
Staffordshire, UK

Matt Griffiths RGN, A&E Cert, FAETC
Senior Nurse, Medicines Management
University Hospitals of Leicester NHS
Trust and
Visiting Professor of Prescribing and
Medicines Management
University of the West of England
Bristol, UK

Jill Hill
Birmingham East and North PCT
Community Diabetes Team Office
Washwood Heath
Birmingham, UK

**Sue Latter PhD, BSc (Hons), RN,
PGDipHV**
Professor of Nursing

School of Health Sciences
University of Southampton
Southampton, UK

Sarah J. O'Brien MB BS, FFPH, DTM&H
School of Transitional Medicine
Clinical Sciences Building
Salford Royal NHS Foundation
Stott Lane
Salford, UK

Barbara Stuttle CBE, MHA, RN, DN, FQNI
Director of Quality and Nursing
Chair, Association for Nurse Prescribing
South West Essex
Basildon
Essex, UK

Tom Walley MD, FRCP, FRCPI
Professor of Clinical Pharmacology
University of Liverpool
Department of Pharmacology and
Therapeutics
Liverpool, UK

**Paul Warburton RN, MSc, CertEd,
ENB 125**
Senior Lecturer and Non-Medical
Prescribing Programme Co-ordinator
Edge Hill University
Faculty of Health
Ormskirk
Lancashire, UK

**Trisha Weller MHS, RGN, NDN Cert,
CPT, DPSCHN(PN)**
Formerly Asthma Lead
Education for Health
Warwick, UK

**Robin Williams MSc, RMN, RGN, CPN
Cert, Dip Nursing (London), IHSM**
Nurse Clinician and Honorary
Lecturer
Department of Pharmacology and
Therapeutics
University of Liverpool
Liverpool, UK

Foreword to the second edition

The extension of the authority to prescribe has moved on apace since the publication of the *Review of the Prescribing, Supply and Administration of Medicines* in 1999. Now nurses, pharmacists, allied health professionals and optometrists, as well as doctors and dentists, can prescribe. These rapid developments have set challenges for professional and regulatory bodies and for individual practitioners. However, all concerned have risen to these challenges with energy and enthusiasm. Training programmes are well developed, many nurses, pharmacists and allied health professionals have completed training, and the benefits to patients are already being felt.

This book is timely and I would like to congratulate Molly Courtenay and Matt Griffiths on bringing together a group of distinguished contributors who have produced an authoritative and comprehensive account of all aspects of prescribing. I am sure that it will prove invaluable both as a practical guide to new prescribers and as a continuing reference source.

I hope that this book will not be seen only as a book for the new prescribing professions. Its thorough examination of all aspects of the prescribing process and the implications of extended prescribing for multidisciplinary teams should also commend it to existing prescribers. It is a valuable text for every professional who is learning to prescribe or who wishes to improve their practice.

I have no doubt that *Independent and Supplementary Prescribing* will inform and support prescribers and that it will make an important contribution to improvements in both the quality and accessibility of patient care.

Dr June Crown CBE

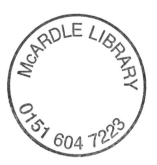

Preface to the second edition

The introduction of non-medical prescribing has meant that nurses, pharmacists, allied health professionals and optometrists have had to expand their practice and so acquire new knowledge and skills in a number of fields. This new knowledge has had to be applied to the many issues surrounding prescribing in the practice setting. There are currently few books available that provide these prescribers with information to help them in this role. As the number of non-medical prescribers grows and as other healthcare professionals take on this role, the need for such information will increase. This book is aimed at those non-medical professions involved in prescribing medicines.

Chapter 1 provides a general overview of non-medical prescribing and describes the current education and training available for extended independent and supplementary prescribers. Chapters 2 to 5 examine non-medical prescribing within a multiprofessional team context, the different models of consultation that might be used by prescribers and the legal and ethical aspects surrounding prescribing. The psychology and sociology of prescribing, applied pharmacology and monitoring skills are explored in chapters 6 to 8. Chapters 9 to 12 deal with promoting concordance, evidence-based prescribing, prescribing within a public health context and the calculation skills required by prescribers. Chapter 13 describes how prescribing can be implemented for practitioners working in the area of dermatology. It is hoped that insights gained from this chapter can be applied to other practice settings. The concluding chapter, chapter 14, examines prescribing errors, their causes and actions to be taken to minimise the risk of prescribing error.

Each chapter is fully referenced and, where appropriate, readers are offered suggestions for further reading and other information sources. We hope that this book will make a positive contribution in a very important aspect of patient care.

Chapter

1

Non-medical prescribing: an overview

Molly Courtenay and Matt Griffiths

In 1986, recommendations were made for nurses to take on the role of prescribing. The Cumberlege report, *Neighbourhood nursing: a focus for care* (Department of Health and Social Security (DHSS) 1986), examined the care given to clients in their homes by district nurses (DNs) and health visitors (HVs). It was identified that some very complicated procedures had arisen around prescribing in the community and that nurses were wasting their time requesting prescriptions from the general practitioner (GP) for such items as wound dressings and ointments. The report suggested that patient care could be improved and resources used more effectively if community nurses were able to prescribe as part of their everyday nursing practice, from a limited list of items and simple agents agreed by the DHSS.

Following the publication of this report, the recommendations for prescribing and its implications were examined. An advisory group was set up by the Department of Health (DoH) to examine nurse prescribing (DoH 1989). Dr June Crown was the Chair of this group.

The following is taken from the Crown report:

> Nurses in the community take a central role in caring for patients in their homes. Nurses are not, however, able to write prescriptions for the products that are needed for patient care, even when the nurse is effectively taking professional responsibility for some aspects of the management of the patient. However experienced or highly skilled in their own areas of practice, nurses must ask a doctor to write a prescription. It is well known that in practice a doctor often rubber stamps a prescribing decision taken by a nurse. This can lead to a lack of clarity about professional responsibilities, and is demeaning to both nurses and doctors. There is wide agreement that action is now needed to align prescribing powers with professional responsibility (DoH 1989).

The report made a number of recommendations involving the categories of items which nurses might prescribe, together with the circumstances under which they might be prescribed. It was recommended that:

> Suitably qualified nurses working in the community should be able, in clearly defined circumstances, to prescribe from a limited list of items and to adjust the timing and dosage of medicines within a set protocol (DoH 1989).

The Crown report identified several groups of patients that would benefit from nurse prescribing. These patients included: patients with a catheter or a stoma; patients suffering with postoperative wounds; and homeless families not registered with a GP. The report also suggested that a number of other benefits would occur as a result of nurses adopting the role of prescriber. As well as improved patient care, these included improved use of both nurses' and patients' time and improved communication between team members arising as a result of a clarification of professional responsibilities (DoH 1989).

During 1992, the primary legislation permitting nurses to prescribe a limited range of drugs was passed (Medicinal Products: Prescription by Nurses etc. Act 1992). The necessary amendments were made to this Act in 1994 and a revised list of products available to the nurse prescriber was published in the *Nurse Prescribers' Formulary* (NPF 2009). In 1994, eight demonstration sites were set up in England for nurse prescribing. By the spring of 2001, approximately 20 000 DNs and HVs were qualified independent prescribers and post-registration programmes for DNs and HVs included the necessary educational component qualifying nurses to prescribe. Later extensions (Nursing and Midwifery Council (NMC) 2005; 2007a) enabled any community nurse (including those without a specialist practitioner qualification) to prescribe from this formulary.

The available research exploring independent nurse prescribing by DNs and HVs indicates that patients are as satisfied, and sometimes more satisfied, with a nurse prescribing as they are with their GP. The quality of the relationship that the nurse has with the patient, the accessibility and approachability of the nurse, the style of consultation and information provided, and the expertise of the nurse are attributes of nurse prescribing viewed positively by patients (Luker et al. 1998). Nurse prescribing enables doctors and nurses to use their time more effectively and treatments are more conveniently provided (Brooks et al. 2001). Time savings and convenience (with regards to not seeing a GP to supply a prescription) are benefits reported by nurses adopting the role of prescriber (Luker et al. 1997). Furthermore, nurses are of the opinion that they provide the patient with better information about their treatment and have reported an increased sense of satisfaction, status and autonomy (Luker et al. 1997; Rodden 2001).

A further report by Crown, which reviewed the prescribing, supply and administration of medicines, was published in 1999 (DoH 1999). The review recommended that prescribing authority should be extended to other groups of professionals with training and expertise in specialist areas. During 2001, support was given by the Government for this extension (DoH 2001). Funding was made available for other nurses, as well as those currently qualified to prescribe, to undergo the necessary training to enable them to prescribe from an extended formulary.

This formulary included:

- A number of specified Prescription Only Medicines (POMs), enabling nurses to prescribe for a number of conditions listed within four treatment areas: minor ailments; minor injuries; health promotion; and palliative care.
- General Sales List (GSL) items, i.e. those that can be sold to the public without the supervision of a pharmacist, used to treat these conditions.
- Pharmacy (P) medicines, i.e. those products sold under the supervision of a pharmacist, used to treat these conditions.

A number of medicines and conditions were added to this formulary between 2003 and 2005 (including medicines for emergency and first contact care) until in 2006 legislation was passed (DoH 2005) enabling nurses to independently prescribe any licensed medicines for any condition within their area of competence and a number of controlled drugs.

Independent prescribing for pharmacists was introduced in 2006 (DoH 2005) and in 2009, further changes in legislation enabled nurse and pharmacist independent prescribers to prescribe unlicensed medicines for their patients and also to mix medicines themselves or direct others to do so (Medicines and Healthcare products Regulatory Agency (MHRA) 2009). At the time of publication of this book, restrictions around controlled drug (CD) prescribing for nurses and pharmacists were still in place. However, lifting of these restrictions is imminent, which will enable nurses and pharmacists to prescribe virtually any CD.

Independent prescribing for optometrists was introduced in 2007 (DoH 2007). Optometrists are able to prescribe any ophthalmic medication for any eye condition within their area of competence.

Supplementary prescribing

The introduction of a new form of prescribing for professions allied to medicine was suggested in 1999 (DoH 1999). It was proposed that this new form of prescribing, i.e. 'dependent prescribing', would take place after a diagnosis had been made by a doctor and a Clinical Management Plan (CMP) drawn up for the patient. The term 'dependent prescribing' has since been superseded by 'supplementary prescribing'.

Supplementary prescribing is 'a voluntary prescribing partnership between an independent prescriber (doctor) and a supplementary prescriber (SP) (nurse or pharmacist) to implement an agreed patient-specific CMP with the patient's agreement' (DoH 2002). Patients with long-term medical conditions such as asthma, diabetes or coronary heart disease, or those with long-term health needs such as anticoagulation therapy, are most likely to benefit from this type of prescribing.

Unlike independent prescribing, there are no legal restrictions on the clinical conditions for which SPs are able to prescribe. Supplementary prescribers are able to prescribe:

- All GSL and P medicines, appliances and devices, foods and other borderline substances approved by the Advisory Committee on Borderline Substances.
- All POMs (including CDs).
- 'Off-label' medicines (medicines for use outside their licensed indications), 'black triangle' drugs and drugs marked 'less suitable for prescribing' in the British National Formulary (BNF).

Unlicensed drugs may only be prescribed if they are part of a clinical trial with a clinical trial certificate or exemption (this may change following proposals set out by the MHRA (MHRA 2004) enabling SPs to prescribe unlicensed medicines).

Training for supplementary prescribing was introduced in 2003 for nurses and pharmacists (DoH 2002) and in 2005 for optometrists and allied health professionals (AHPs), i.e. physiotherapists, podiatrists/chiropodists and radiographers (DoH 2005).

Training is based on that for independent prescribing. The taught element of the course is 26/27 days, of which a substantial proportion is face-to-face contact time, although other ways of learning, such as open and distance learning (DL) formats, might be used. Students are also required to undertake additional self-directed learning and 12/13 days learning in practice with a medical prescriber.

Training for independent prescribing is now combined with that for SP in all higher education institutions (HEIs). The Royal Pharmaceutical Society of Great Britain (RPSGB 2003), which is responsible for validating SP programmes for pharmacists, has acknowledged that as 60–70% of the SP curriculum will be common to both nurses and pharmacists, institutions running the SP curriculum for nurses provide an ideal opportunity for shared learning. A number of HEIs run the combined independent/supplementary prescribing programme for nurses, pharmacists and AHPs. Nurses and pharmacists qualify as both independent and supplementary prescribers and AHPs as supplementary prescribers.

Educational preparation for extended prescribers

An outline curriculum for the educational preparation for independent prescribing was produced by the English National Board (ENB) in September 2001 (ENB 2006). Following the closure of the ENB, the NMC has continued to apply the ENB's existing standards and guidance for the approval of HEIs with regards to registerable and recordable programmes. Standards of proficiency for nurse and midwife prescribers were published in 2006 (NMC 2006).

A number of prerequisites are required by those who wish to undertake independent and supplementary prescribing training. These include:

- Registration with the NMC as a first level nurse or midwife or, for pharmacists, current registration with the RPSGB and/or the Pharmaceutical Society of Northern Ireland (PSNI). AHPs must be registered with the Health Professions Council in one of the relevant allied health professions legally able to prescribe.
- The ability to study at level 3 (degree level).
- At least three years' experience as a qualified nurse (the year immediately preceding application to the programme must be in the clinical field in which the candidate wishes to prescribe). For pharmacists, the level of relevant knowledge and expertise is dependent upon the nature of their practice and the length of their experience. AHPs must normally have at least three years of post-qualification experience.
- Agreement from a doctor that they will contribute to the 12/13 days learning in practice (including the assessment process), and post-qualifying experience.
- Employer's agreement to undertake the course and also that they will support continuing professional development (CPD).
- Commitment by their employer to enable access to prescribing budgets and other necessary arrangements for prescribing in practice.
- Occupation of a post in which they are expected to prescribe.

Nurses, pharmacists and AHPs must also be assessed by their employer as competent to take a history, and make a clinical assessment and diagnosis. Nurses and AHPs must also demonstrate appropriate numeracy skills.

The independent and supplementary prescribing training programme involves at least 26 days in the classroom (for distance learning programmes, eight taught days must be included in the programme) and 12 days in practice with a designated medical practitioner. Courses generally run over three to six months, but must be completed within one year. Topics taught include:

- Consultation skills.
- Influences on the psychology of prescribing.
- Prescribing in a team context.
- Clinical pharmacology.
- Evidence-based practice.

- Legal, policy and ethical aspects.
- Professional accountability and responsibility.
- Prescribing in the public health context.

A range of assessments are used to assess students' knowledge and skills including a numeracy assessment in which a 100% pass rate must be achieved. In addition, nurses are required to demonstrate that they are aware of the anatomical and physiological difference between children and adults, are able to take an appropriate history and clinical assessment, and can make an appropriate decision to diagnose or refer (NMC 2007b).

Nurse prescribers are not required to undertake any additional hours of practice to meet CPD needs. However, appraisal of these needs should be undertaken on a yearly basis as part of performance review, and support to meet these needs must be provided by the nurse prescriber's employer (NMC 2008).

The combined independent and supplementary prescribing programme varies with regards to Credit Accumulation and Transfer (CAT) points awarded but is generally between 20 and 40 CAT points. In a number of universities and HEIs the prescribing module has been incorporated into post-qualification pathways such as the nurse practitioner course. In some of these instances, the number of academic credits are available at masters level.

For further discussion of supplementary prescribing see chapter 2.

Conclusion

The initial development of non-medical prescribing was slow. It was first considered by the Government for nurses in 1986 and the first formulary for DNs and HVs was extremely limited. Between 2002 and 2006 policy changes were rapid and nurses and pharmacists now have virtually the same prescribing rights as doctors. Although AHPs are currently restricted to supplementary prescribing, future policy changes will probably see the extension of independent prescribing rights to this group and the extension of supplementary prescribing to other healthcare professionals.

The delivery of healthcare within the United Kingdom is constantly changing. In order to ensure the survival of the National Health Service, and the development of future services, the skills of practitioners must be used appropriately. This means that where practitioners have the knowledge and skills with regards to the adoption of roles such as prescribing, and patients are happy with the services these practitioners are able to provide, they must be given the opportunity to do so.

References

Brooks, N., Otway, C., Rashid, C., Kilty, E., Maggs, C. (2001). The patients' view: the benefits and limitations of nurse prescribing. *British Journal of Community Nursing* 6(7): 342–348.

DHSS (1986). *Neighbourhood Nursing: a Focus for Care (Cumberlege Report)*. London: HMSO.

DoH (1989). *Report of the Advisory Group on Nurse Prescribing (Crown Report)*. London: DoH.

DoH (1999). *Review of Prescribing, Supply and Administration of Medicines (Crown Report)*. London: DoH.

DoH (2001). *Patients to get Quicker Access to Medicines (Press Release)*. London: DoH.

DoH (2002). *Supplementary Prescribing*. London: DoH.

DoH (2005). *Written ministerial statement on the expansion of independent nurse prescribing and introduction of pharmacists independent prescribing*. London: DoH.

DoH (2007). *Optometrists to get Independent Prescribing Rights (Press Release)*. London: DoH.

Luker, K., Austin, L., Ferguson, B., Smith, K. (1997). Nurse prescribing: the views of nurses and other health care professionals. *British Journal of Community Health Nursing* 2: 69–74.

Luker, K.A., Austin, L., Hogg, C., Ferguson, B., Smith, K. (1998). Nurse-patient relationships: the context of nurse prescribing. *Journal of Advanced Nursing* 28(2): 235–242.

MHRA (2004). *Supplementary Prescribing: Use of Unlicensed Medicines, Reformulation of Licensed Products and Preparations made from Active Pharmaceutical Ingredients and Exipients*. London: MHRA.

MHRA (2009). *Revised statement on medical and non-medical prescribing and mixing medicines in clinical practice*. London: MHRA.

NMC (2005). V100 nurse prescribers. Circular 30/2005 (SAT/1P).

NMC (2006). *Standards of proficiency for nurse and midwife prescribers*. London: NMC.

NMC (2007a). Standards of educational preparation for prescribing from the community NPF for nurses without a specialist practice qualification. V150.

NMC (2007b). Prescribing for children and young people. Circular 22/2007.

NMC (2008). Guidance for CPD for nurse and midwife prescribers. Circular 10/2008.

Nurse Prescribers' Formulary for Community Practitioners (NPF) (2009). London: British Medical Association and Royal Pharmaceutical Society of Great Britain.

Rodden, C., (2001). Nurse prescribing: views on autonomy and independence. *British Journal of Community Nursing* 6(7): 350–355.

RPSGB (2003). Outline curriculum for training programmes to prepare pharmacist supplementary prescribers. www.rpsgb.org.uk

Non-medical prescribing in a multidisciplinary team context

Barbara Stuttle

The demands by patients for a more streamlined, accessible and flexible service (Department of Health (DoH) 2000), demands for the integration of services (DoH 2008) and a high-quality accountable service, and demands for roles which extend beyond traditional boundaries acknowledging the range of knowledge and skills held by practitioners and offering them the opportunity to achieve their full potential (DoH 2001; 2002), have meant that the roles of healthcare professionals have changed dramatically over recent years. These changes have placed a great emphasis on teamwork and multiprofessional co-operation.

The success of non-medical prescribing is dependent upon the contributions from a number of practitioners, including specialist nurses, pharmacists and doctors, and the ability of these professionals to work together as a team. This chapter examines the key issues that need to be considered by healthcare professionals if non-medical prescribing is to be implemented effectively. It commences with an exploration of teamwork and then moves on to discuss clinical governance. Communication, sharing information and supplementary prescribing are then examined.

Teamwork

In order to work effectively as a team, a number of key elements are required. These include:

- Effective verbal and written communication.
- Enabling and encouraging supervision.
- Collaboration and common goals.
- Valuing the contributions of team members and matching team roles to ability.
- A culture that encourages team members to seek help.
- Team structure (Vincent et al. 1998).

Underpinning each of the above elements is the need for team members to have a clear understanding of one another's roles and the ability to communicate with one another. As non-medical prescribing has changed the role boundaries of professions allied to medicine, so the roles and relationships between healthcare professionals have changed. For example, the nurse adopting the role of prescriber affects the role of the pharmacist. The conversations surrounding medicines that once took place between the pharmacist and the doctor now take place between the pharmacist, doctor and nurse.

Conversely, it is important that the nurse is aware of the support the pharmacist is able to provide. This support will vary depending upon the environment within which the pharmacist works. If the pharmacist is working in a hospital setting and as a member of the ward team, they will have greater information about the patient's conditions and specific problems. The role of the pharmacist is therefore enhanced. As well as the interpretation of prescriptions, checking drug dosage levels and monitoring prescriptions for possible drug interactions, they may well be able to advise colleagues on a number of topics in relation to drug therapy, undertake medication reviews, discharge planning, education and training (Downie et al. 2003). Furthermore, with the introduction of independent and supplementary prescribing for pharmacists, pharmacists may well be leading clinics, such as anticoagulation or pain control clinics, and so be able to provide the nurse with a greater wealth of information and be an extremely useful resource in all aspects of prescribing and medicines management.

Another area in which confusion may occur, if roles are not fully understood, is levels of competency. For example, the ability of a nurse to prescribe means that they are able to carry out a complete episode of care. However, not all nurses within a team are qualified to prescribe. Therefore, there may be a lack of consistency or continuity of care if other non-prescribing nurses care for the patient. Unless these different levels of competency with regards to prescribing are understood between team members, this could result in inequity of service and confusion for the patient. It also needs to be clear who directs the care for the patient.

The advent of non-medical prescribing has therefore emphasised the need to clarify the activity of team members, i.e. those activities common to some professions, and those specific to the role of one discipline only. It has been suggested that without this clarity, team members might drift towards common ground and some areas of practice could become neglected (McCray 2002).

The core values of multidisciplinary work have been described as trust and sharing (Loxley 1997). An essential component of these values is that trust and sharing are a two-way process. Not only does the team rely on the individual's commitment to the task, but members must take on the team's belief in themselves and meet their expectations. If members of the team are to trust one another and share their experiences, confidence and a clear understanding of one's own professional role is essential (Loxley 1997).

For example, nurses have traditionally been seen as semi-autonomous practitioners working within the guidelines set by doctors. Medical staff have been seen as those making autonomous decisions and advising on practice. Some professions allied to medicine, e.g. physiotherapists, although practising autonomously, work primarily on an individual basis with clients. It is suggested by McCray (2002) that power and status, as a result of these differences, may well become an issue and influence trust and sharing when working together in a team. Doctors may well find it difficult to take advice from some healthcare professionals. By contrast, nurses may not feel confident enough to provide advice in relation to their own area of practice.

Clinical governance

Clinical governance has been defined as:

> A framework through which NHS organisations are accountable for continually improving the quality of their services and safeguarding high standards of care by creating an environment to which excellence in clinical care will flourish (Scally and Donaldson 1998).

Clinical governance has been responsible for bringing professionals together as a multi-professional team, to collaborate and learn from each other. This has meant moving away from a culture of self-protection and blame, to one where self-regulation and learning through experience are valued (Jasper 2002). By working together and reflecting on the skills and knowledge of team members, the opportunities for progress and improvement in patient care are immense. The Bristol Royal Infirmary Inquiry (doh.gov.uk/bristolinquiry) and Victoria Climbie (http://www.victoria-climbie-inquiry.org.uk/finreport/finreport.html) provide examples of where teamwork and communication broke down. Recommendations from these reports focus on team working, communication, sharing information and joint learning.

Drug therapy is becoming increasingly complex. Many patients receive multiple drugs and therefore the possibility of error while administering medicines is large. An error that involves the administration of a drug can be a disaster for the patient. Drug administration generally involves several members of the multidisciplinary team and will include a chain of events involving several people, i.e. the manufacturer, distributor, pharmacist, prescriber, hospital managers and patient. A number of errors that may occur at each level have been identified by Downie et al. (2003). These include:

Prescriber error:

Poor handwriting.

Abbreviations.

Confusion of product names that look similar.

Omission of essential information.

Pharmacist error:

Error in labelling medicines.

Supply of medicines to wards without information on the actions, dose and use of the product.

Lack of withdrawal of a product due to a fault, i.e. there is a need for rapid communication from pharmaceutical staff to ward staff.

Lack of information about a product which is part of a clinical trial. If information is not supplied to ward staff involved in the trial, the product may not be used safely.

Error by the nurse administering the medicine:

Misinterpretation of the prescription.

Selection of the incorrect medicine to be administered.

Inaccurate record of administration.

Error by the nurse manager:

Lack of up-to-date drug information, i.e. BNF and local formularies unavailable.

No clear lines of communication with clinical pharmacists and Medicines Information Service.

Inappropriate staff members administering medicines.

Inaccurate and illegible records regarding the drugs administered.

Unsafe storage of medicines.

Lack of withdrawal of medicines when no longer required.

No consideration to timing and number of medicine rounds.

Prescribing and recording documents not of the required standard and inappropriate for the area of practice.

Procedures used in the event of a drug error seen as a deterrent by nurses, i.e. a 'blame' culture.

An absence of a multidisciplinary drug and therapeutics committee to review medicines management issues.

Level of risk not assessed, i.e. some drugs more complicated to administer than others.

Patient error:

Lack of co-operation by the patient in order to achieve therapeutic benefits of the drug.

Rejection of treatment by the patient as a result of a lack of understanding (by the patient) about the drug therapy.

Clinical governance is a useful tool which can be used by the multidisciplinary team to maintain and improve the quality of non-medical prescribing and demonstrate that prescribing practice is in the best interests of the patient. It should ensure that each member of the prescribing team, i.e. doctor, nurse and pharmacist, recognises their role in providing high-quality patient care, and how the team can work together to improve prescribing standards.

Regular team meetings provide a forum in which members of the multidisciplinary team can work together to achieve common goals, and develop standards of care and protocols for prescribing. Within these meetings, awareness needs to be raised with regards to such systems as the Yellow Card Scheme for the spontaneous reporting of suspected adverse drug reactions by doctors, dentists, pharmacists, coroners and nurses (medicines.mhra.gov.uk), and the National Patient Safety Agency (NPSA) for reporting drug errors (www.npsa.nhs.uk). The NPSA hope that by promoting a fair and open culture in the NHS, staff will be encouraged to report incidents and so learn from any problems that affect the safety of patients. If team meetings raise staff awareness of the NPSA and errors are discussed, this will enable individuals to reflect and learn from mistakes and to take the appropriate action to prevent them happening again. There will be a move away from a 'blame' culture and patient safety will be increased.

Once standards of care have been set and implemented by members of the multiprofessional team, the team will be able to undertake periodic audits of prescribing practice. The outcome of these audits can be used to identify areas of prescribing practice that require improvement, and also the education and training needs of individuals. All healthcare professionals have a responsibility for their individual professional development and maintenance of prescribing knowledge. By working as a multiprofessional team, the needs of individuals can be identified, education and training programmes accessed, and learning shared across professional boundaries.

Communication and sharing information

The sharing of accurate information between multidisciplinary team members is vitally important. It was highlighted by the Crown report (DoH 1989) that good communication between health professionals and patients, and between different professionals, is essential for high-quality healthcare.

Good record keeping in relation to prescribing is essential and provides an efficient method of communication and dissemination of information between members of the multidisciplinary team. The healthcare record is a tool for communication within the team. It should provide clear evidence of the care planned, the decisions made, the care delivered and the information shared.

The prescription details, together with other details of the consultation with the patient, should be entered into the patient's record. The record should clearly indicate the date, the name of the prescriber, the name of the items prescribed and the quantity prescribed (or dose, frequency and treatment duration) at the time of generating the prescription. Where nurses hold separate nursing records, they have a responsibility to ensure this information is entered into the medical record as soon as possible and preferably contemporaneously. All health professionals qualified to prescribe should have access to the relevant patient records. Ideally, these records should be shared between team members.

Supplementary prescribing and teamwork

Supplementary prescribing is described in chapter 1. The information outlined below can be found at www.doh.gov.uk/supplementaryprescribing. The nature of supplementary prescribing heightens the need for good teamwork. The patient, independent prescriber (IP) and supplementary prescriber (SP) are required to work in partnership to develop the Clinical Management Plan (CMP) (see Figures 2.1 and 2.2). The IP is responsible for the diagnosis and setting the parameters of the CMP, although they need not personally draw it up. The principle underlying the concept of supplementary prescribing must be explained in advance to the patient by the IP or the SP and their agreement should be obtained. The IP and the SP must agree and sign the CMP.

It should also be clear from information recorded on the CMP as to when the plan will be reviewed by the IP. Supplementary prescribing must be supported by a regular clinical review of the patient's progress by the assessing clinician (the IP), at predetermined intervals appropriate to the patient's condition and the medicines to be prescribed. This may be a joint review by both the IP and the SP. Where this is not possible, the IP should review the patient, and subsequently discuss the future management of the patient's conditions(s) with the SP. The intervals should normally be no longer than one year.

Both prescribers must record their agreement to the continuing or amended CMP and the patient's agreement to the continuation of the supplementary prescribing arrangement, in order for the CMP to remain valid. They should set a new review date. Prescribing by the SP should not continue after the date of review without a recorded agreement to the next phase of the CMP.

Discontinuation of supplementary prescribing is at the discretion of the IP. However, this mode of prescribing can also be discontinued at the request of the SP or the patient. Furthermore, where there is a sole IP and he or she is replaced for whatever reason, the CMP must be reviewed by their successor.

In order for effective implementation of supplementary prescribing, the following factors are important:

- It must be simple, i.e. the CMP should not duplicate information already in the shared records.
- The CMP need only make a reference to the appropriate guideline for the treatment of a condition. There is no need to produce lists of medicines.
- Supplementary prescribing must be flexible. The IP and SP will need to work differently in different settings. For example, if the IP and SP are not in close contact, shared electronic records might be required. There may also be a need for team partnerships,

Name of Patient:	Patient medication sensitivities/allergies:
Patient identification e.g. ID number, date of birth:	
Independent Prescriber(s):	Supplementary Prescriber(s)
Condition(s) to be treated	Aim of treatment

Medicines that may be prescribed by SP:

Preparation	Indication	Dose schedule	Specific indications for referral back to the IP
		.	.

Guidelines or protocols supporting Clinical Management Plan:

Frequency of review and monitoring by:

Supplementary prescriber	Supplementary prescriber and independent prescriber

Process for reporting ADRs:

Shared record to be used by IP and SP:

Agreed by independent prescriber(s)	Date	Agreed by supplementary prescriber(s)	Date	Date agreed with patient/carer

Figure 2.1 The CMP (for teams that have full co-terminus access to patient records) (doh.gov.uk/supplementary prescribing)

i.e. the SP may need to form a partnership with more than one IP (www.doh.gov.uk/ supplementaryprescribing).

Interestingly, as the shared care record develops, and electronic records and electronic prescribing are used more widely, particularly in the care of patients with long-term conditions, there will be greater consistency and clarity, which will make the whole process easier to audit.

Name of Patient:	Patient medication sensitivities/allergies:
Patient identification e.g. ID number, date of birth:	
Current medication:	Medical history:
Independent Prescriber(s): Contact details: [tel/email/address]	Supplementary prescriber(s): Contact details: [tel/email/address]
Condition(s) to be treated:	Aim of treatment:

Medicines that may be prescribed by SP:

Preparation	Indication	Dose schedule	Specific indications for referral back to the IP

Guidelines or protocols supporting Clinical Management Plan:

Frequency of review and monitoring by:

Supplementary prescriber	Supplementary prescriber and independent prescriber

Process for reporting ADRs:

Shared record to be used by IP and SP:

Agreed by independent prescriber(s):	Date	Agreed by supplementary prescriber(s):	Date	Date agreed with patient/carer

Figure 2.2 CMP (for teams where the SP does not have co-terminus access to the medical record) (doh.gov.uk/supplementary prescribing)

Conclusion

Non-medical prescribing is a success and it is widely used in care provision. It is important that those healthcare professionals involved in prescribing develop good relationships with one another. This will lead to trust, confidence, respect, the sharing of information and a clear understanding of one another's roles. This will enable individuals to work together effectively as a team ensuring high-quality, consistent care is provided to patients.

Clinical governance is a useful tool that should be used by the multiprofessional team in order to maintain and improve the quality of non-medical prescribing. Clinical governance standards should be high and regularly monitored at the highest level within organisations. Quality is a key aspect of all healthcare and the rigour that clinical governance provides is an easy framework in which non-medical prescribers should work. However, within this framework, teamwork is essential.

References

DoH (1989). *Report of the Advisory Group on Nurse Prescribing (Crown report)*. London: DoH.

DoH (2000). *A Health Service of All the Talents: Developing the NHS Workforce*. London: DoH.

DoH (2001). *Essence of Care*. London: DoH.

DoH (2002). *Liberating the Talents*. London: The Stationery Office.

DoH (2008). *High Quality Care for All: NHS Next Stage Review Final Report*. London: DoH.

Downie, G., Mackenzie, J., Williams, A. (2003). *Pharmacology and Medicines Management for Nurses* (third edition). London: Churchill Livingstone.

Jasper, M. (2002). Challenges to professional practice. In: Hogston, R., Simpson, P. *Foundations of Nursing Practice*. Basingstoke: Palgrave Macmillan.

Loxley, A. (1997). *Collaboration in Health and Welfare*. London: Jessica Kingsley.

McCray, J. (2002). Nursing practice in an interprofessional context. In: Hogston, R., Simpson, P. *Foundations of Nursing Practice*. Basingstoke: Palgrave Macmillan.

Scally, G., Donaldson, L.J. (1998). Clinical governance and the drive for quality improvement in the new NHS in England. *British Medical Journal 317*: 61–65.

Vincent, C.A., Adams, S., Stanhope, N. (1998). A framework for the analysis of risk and safety in medicines. *British Medical Journal 316*: 1154–1157.

Consultation skills and decision making

Anne Baird

Much of the research on the consultation has developed from the desire of general practice to carve out for itself a specific body of expertise distinct from hospital medicine (Drucquer and Hutchinson 2000). As a result, while there is a considerable amount of literature relating to general practice, as practised by the general practitioner (GP), little has been written on consultations by other health professionals, and little on consultations in secondary care. This chapter will endeavour to introduce to the reader some of the key texts on consultation models and communication skills, and discuss their relevance for non-medical prescribers. Patients' health beliefs will be briefly explored, as will the literature comparing the outcomes of consultations by doctors and other health professionals. Decision-making strategies and diagnosis will be looked at, with a brief overview of computer decision support in the consultation. A chapter such as this can only hope to give a brief synopsis of these issues, and it is hoped that the reader will use the reference list to follow-up areas of particular interest in more detail.

Consultation models

The concept of nurses and other healthcare professionals (HCPs) undertaking a consultation is relatively new. While the consultation will for many prescribers form the basis of the interaction during which they prescribe, for others, this will be less clear... consider ward-based practitioners and those working in the patient's home. However, for practitioners working in all of these settings, many of the concepts discussed will be of relevance. It is interesting to note that while GP registrars are extensively trained and heavily assessed in consultation skills, other practitioners new to consulting may be given little or no support in gaining these skills. While they are able to draw on the communication skills they have always made use of, applying these within a different context can bring difficulties. The emphasis given to the consultation in the prescribing course will provide a valuable opportunity for many practitioners to examine and improve their skills in this area. A useful tool with which to analyse one's own consultation is the CAIIN model (Consultation Assessment and Improvement Instrument for Nurses) (Hastings and Redsell 2006). Though aimed at nurses, it encompasses both primary and secondary care perspectives and is a useful resource for anyone seeking to develop their consulting skills.

So, what are consultation models and do they have any practical applications? The best known models, which are discussed below, can be described as either normative (what should happen in a consultation) or descriptive (what does happen in a consultation).

Byrne and Long (1976)

One of the first examples of a descriptive model is that of Byrne and Long (1976), which is based on an analysis of over 2000 recorded consultations. They identified six phases to the consultation:

- Phase I. The doctor establishes a relationship with the patient.
- Phase II. The doctor attempts to discover, or does discover, the reason for the patient's attendance.
- Phase III. The doctor conducts a verbal or physical examination or both.
- Phase IV. The doctor, or the doctor and the patient, or the patient (in that order of probability) consider the condition.
- Phase V. The doctor, and occasionally the patient, detail further treatment or further investigation.
- Phase VI. The consultation is terminated, usually by the doctor.
- (Phase VII. The 'parting shot'.)

In reality, consultations rarely unfold in such a logical manner, though all phases are likely to occur at some stage (including, possibly, the 'parting shot' when the patient reveals the real reason for their attendance just as they are about to leave!). Byrne and Long (1976) noted that, unsurprisingly, consultations are likely to go wrong if there are shortcomings in phase II (there is a failure to discover the reason for attending) or phase IV (there is a failure to adequately consider the implications of the problem). They also noted that, on average, doctors interrupted patients within 18 seconds of the start of the consultation.

Stott and Davies (1979)

Stott and Davies' model identified four areas which could potentially be explored within each consultation. These are:

- Management of the presenting problem. This is key, and if not dealt with, the patient is unlikely to be receptive to any other activities.
- Modification of help-seeking behaviours. This could include, for example, a discussion on how to manage a sore throat at home in the future.
- Review of long-term problems, for example, a blood pressure check.
- Opportunistic health promotion, for example, mentioning overdue cervical cytology or a discussion of smoking cessation.

Pendleton et al. (1984)

Pendleton et al. are best known for their discussion of the patient's **ideas, concerns** and **expectations**, and the concept of a patient-centred, rather than a doctor-centred, consultation. They detail seven tasks of the consultation. By now, similar themes are beginning to emerge from each of the models.

1. To define the reason for attendance, including:
    - The nature/history of the problem.
    - Aetiology.
    - The patient's ideas, concerns and expectations.
    - The effects of the problem.

2. To consider other problems:
   - Continuing problems.
   - Risk factors.
3. With the patient, to choose an appropriate action for each problem.
4. To achieve a shared understanding of the problem with the patient.
5. To involve the patient in the management and encourage him or her to accept appropriate responsibility.
6. To use time and resources appropriately.
7. To establish and maintain a relationship.

This model is one in which the practitioner works in partnership with the patient to find a solution satisfactory to both. For example, a mother bringing her child to surgery with a possible ear infection may believe that antibiotics are necessary as they have previously been prescribed. Furthermore, she may believe that she would be negligent not to bring the child. Or the manager consulting with a sore throat may be anxious that he will be unable to deliver an important presentation next week. If the practitioner is able to acknowledge the importance to the patient of these concerns, it is more likely that a solution acceptable to both parties will be reached.

Factors 6 and 7 deal with concerns outwith the immediate consultation, but nonetheless important. An awareness of the finite nature of resources (e.g. time or money), and wisdom in their use, is essential for the wellbeing of the practitioner as well as the patient. The establishing of a relationship, either for the duration of the consultation or which may be ongoing for many years, is also important for patient and practitioner satisfaction.

Neighbour (1987)

Roger Neighbour, in his most readable book, builds on the other models in his view of the consultation as a journey with 'checkpoints' along the way.

- Connecting. This first checkpoint is to do with establishing a relationship and building a rapport with the patient, and is identified by Neighbour as the first essential task of the consultation.
- Summarising. The second checkpoint includes taking a history, summarising the problem and reflecting it back to the patient to ensure there are no misunderstandings. It also involves considering the patient's ideas, concerns and expectations.
- Handing over. By this time, the practitioner will have brought the consultation to a point where the patient and the practitioner's agendas have been agreed and dealt with, and a management plan developed.
- Safety netting. This involves acknowledging that things may not turn out as planned, and ensuring that the patient knows what to do should this happen. It may involve sharing with the patient some of the other possible diagnoses and outcomes. For example, the patient with asthma could be advised to increase use of their bronchodilator inhaler, but to monitor their peak flow and to return if their peak flow continues to fall.
- Housekeeping. This is where the practitioner looks to themselves and their response to the consultation. It may involve having a brief chat with a colleague over a coffee or merely acknowledging to oneself the effect a particular consultation has had.

Calgary–Cambridge model (1998)

More recently, Silverman et al. (1998) have explored the consultation in considerable depth, through an approach which has become known as the Calgary–Cambridge model (so named because of its origins in the University of Calgary, Canada and the University of Cambridge, UK). They build upon the body of knowledge referred to in other well-known models. An outline plan of their model is described below, but readers are advised to consult the book for a more detailed study of their method.

1. Initiating the session.
   - Establishing initial rapport.
   - Involving the patient.
2. Gathering information.
   - Exploration of problems.
   - Understanding the patient's perspective.
   - Providing structure to the consultation.
3. Building the relationship.
   - Developing rapport.
   - Involving the patient.
4. Explanation and planning.
   - Providing the correct amount and type of information.
   - Aiding accurate recall and understanding.
   - Achieving a shared understanding.
   - Planning – shared decision making.
5. Closing the session.

The work of Silverman et al. builds on the strong body of research into the consultation which precedes it, some of which has been discussed above. Again, similar themes are explored. The concept of the patient's agenda is prominent, while the value of providing structure to the consultation is stressed. It can be reassuring to realise that a patient-centred consultation does not mean that the practitioner abdicates all responsibility to the patient. Rather, both patient and practitioner will feel more secure if the practitioner is able to give some structure and direction to the consultation, while addressing the patient's concerns.

Silverman et al. also address specifically the issue of closing the session, something which nurses may find difficult, possibly because of the perception of many patients that nurses are more approachable and have more time than doctors. Suggestions include agreeing on specific follow-up and setting another appointment. Tate (2003) goes a step further in suggesting that standing up and holding the door open may be required! Personally, I have sometimes found it necessary to help particularly garrulous patients into their coats and gently guide them through the door!

Communication skills

Consultation models are helpful but without the use of appropriate skills on the part of the practitioner, they remain sterile. Much of the literature on consultation models also discusses the skills needed for an effective consultation. It has been shown that good communication skills on the part of the practitioner greatly affect the outcome of the consultation. Maguire and Pitceathly (2002) suggest that doctors with good consultation skills identify patients' problems more accurately. Patients are more satisfied with the care they receive and leave the consultation with a better understanding of their problems, proposed investigations and treatment options. They are more likely to adhere to treatment and lifestyle changes, and distress and anxiety are lessened. An added bonus would appear to be increased wellbeing and satisfaction for the practitioner.

Communication skills are included in nurses' core training, but this does not mean that they can afford to be complacent. Chant et al. (2002), in a literature review, has suggested that this training may at times be lacking and that there is a wide variation in the quality of nurse/patient communication. While Bond et al. (1999) found that trainee nurse practitioners rated uniformly highly in consultation skills, another study by Greco and Powell (2002) suggests that although this is generally true, it is by no means always the case.

Which communication skills are required for an effective consultation? What follows is of necessity a brief overview; readers are directed to more comprehensive texts for a more thorough examination of the topic. Silverman et al. (1998) have identified a total of 72 skills which can be used within the consultation and most of the literature on consultation models also examines the necessary skills.

The consultation skills needed by the prescriber are no different to those used in other aspects of practice. An appropriate environment, i.e. one which supports privacy and confidentiality, is important (While 2002), and may pose particular challenges for ward-based prescribers and those working in the patient's home. Strategies to support the patient in telling their story include open and closed questioning, active listening and the appropriate use of eye contact and other body language. The recent interest in narrative-based medicine (Launer 2002), where the telling of the patient's story is central to the consultation, draws heavily upon the skills used in family therapy.

Central to the success of the consultation is the ability of the practitioner to identify what the patient hopes to get out of the consultation – i.e. their ideas, concerns and expectations (Pendleton et al. 1984). Research has shown that many patients find it difficult to voice their true concerns (Barry et al. 2000), leading the authors to suggest that patients are not 'fully present' in the consultation. This failure in communication may contribute to inappropriate prescribing decisions; for example, the doctor may prescribe and the patient may take medicine, both just for the sake of the relationship (Britten et al. 2000). There has been a tendency for doctors to assume that patients consult for the sake of a prescription, whereas on many occasions, they may prefer advice or simply be seeking reassurance (Barry et al. 2000; Britten et al. 2000). Consultations with other practitioners have to some extent been free of this preconception until recently, and non-medical prescribers will need to take care to ensure that they continue to reserve the prescription only for those situations where it is genuinely required.

The patient's health beliefs

Stewart and Roter (1989) have discussed in their disease–illness model an analysis of the different perspectives of patient and practitioner for the sickness they are dealing with. According to this model, 'disease' is the cause of sickness in terms of pathophysiology, while 'illness' is the patient's unique experience of sickness. Patients can experience illness but have no disease; for example, the many patients who present in general practice complaining of tiredness for which no organic cause can be found. Similarly, patients may have a disease without experiencing illness; for example, the patient with hypertension is likely to feel completely well. Similar diseases may cause a widely varying illness experience in different individuals, due to their concerns, expectation, support systems and previous experiences (Silverman et al. 1998). This theory goes some way to explain why one individual may consult for an episode of ill health (e.g. a sore throat) whereas another is quite happy to let nature take its course. Traditionally, doctors have confined themselves to seeking out underlying disease, but this perspective is narrower than that of the patient and may lead to an unsatisfactory conclusion.

Patients' illness experience depends to a great extent upon their perspective on their health. Rotter's locus of control theory and Rosenstock's health belief model (Kemm and Close 1995) go some way to explaining why patients have such widely varying health experiences, and are discussed briefly below.

Many readers will be familiar with the concept of the locus of control (Rotter 1954), which is concerned with the extent to which an individual feels able to influence and control their own life. According to this theory, people's health beliefs fall into three broad categories:

- Internal locus of control. These individuals tend to believe that they are responsible for their own health and that what happens to them is the result of their own actions. They will tend to like explanations and discussion, and will want to be involved in decision making about their health.

- External locus of control. Those with an external locus of control tend to have a fatalistic attitude to life and health, and will be reluctant to make changes as they believe that their future is mapped out and there is nothing to be done about it.

- The powerful other. These people will tend to see the responsibility for their health as lying with other people, such as health professionals. They will be reluctant to take responsibility for their own health and are most happy with an authoritarian approach.

Of course, these are broad categories, and most people will lie somewhere along the continuum. They may well espouse different belief systems for different areas of their lives. Tate (2003) suggests that an awareness of where an individual's locus of control lies can help the practitioner to adopt the most appropriate skills.

Another well–known model is Rosenstock's health belief model (1974). He suggests that an individual's motivation to take action is dependent upon four factors:

- Perceived vulnerability. For example, those who believe that they are likely to develop lung cancer are more likely to heed advice to stop smoking that those who do not believe that they are at risk.

- Perceived seriousness. Hypertension may not be regarded as a serious condition to some people, as it does not cause them to feel unwell. However, to the woman who has just lost her mother to a stroke it may seem very serious.

- Perceived benefits. People will weigh up the advantages and disadvantages of a particular course of action. To the individual with high blood pressure, the side effects of the treatment may seem to outweigh any supposed benefit.

- Perceived barriers. These are various barriers a person would need to overcome to go along with the suggested course of action, including physical, psychological and financial. To the person unconvinced of the need to treat high blood pressure, the financial implications of the prescription charge may prove to be the final disincentive.

An awareness of these factors may help the practitioner to understand the patient's particular anxieties and to tailor their interventions accordingly.

Consultations with nurses

Much of the literature comparing consultations by nurses and doctors examines the outcomes of the consultation, rather than the process of consulting. Most of it also relates to a general practice setting, in particular that of nurses running minor illness/first point of contact services. The outcomes do, however, shed some light on the consulting-style favoured by nurses, suggesting that it would tend to be patient-centred rather than practitioner-centred.

Reveley (1998), in an analysis of the role of the triage nurse in general practice, suggests that patients value the caring and supportive aspects of consulting with a nurse, the length of time they have with the nurse and the accessibility of the nurse. Many other studies (Horrocks et al. 2002; Kinnersley et al. 2000; Shum et al. 2000) have found greater patient satisfaction with nurse consultations than with GP consultations (although patients report high levels of satisfaction with both). Importantly, they also found no significant difference in other health outcomes – as Tate (2003) pointed out, patient satisfaction is a blunt (if popular) tool with which to measure the success of the consultation. Many patients will be satisfied if they get what they want, even if this does not necessarily represent best clinical practice.

Most of these studies found that consultations with nurses were slightly longer; that nurses gave more information to patients; and that they offered more advice on self-care and self-management. Interestingly, Kinnersley et al. (2000) observed that although nurses gave more advice on self-care, a similar number of patients consulting with the nurse as with the doctor said they would consult again with the same condition. Kinnersley et al. (2000) suggest that this may be because prescribing rates between the doctors and nurses were similar, validating the patient's decision to seek help rather than self-manage.

Most, if not all, of these studies observe that consultations with nurses are longer than consultations with doctors, and it must be asked how many of the improved outcomes relate to this fact alone. Many doctors would argue that they too would achieve higher patient satisfaction rates with longer consultations, and that this is a feature of the length of time rather than of the skills of the practitioner. This is, of course, entirely possible. Interestingly, Reveley (1998) observed that nurse practitioners (NPs) made significantly less referrals to the practice nurse (PN) than did GPs (5.6% for the NPs; 29% for the GPs). Although the reasons for these referrals is not explored, it may be that they were for investigations (e.g. blood tests) or treatments (e.g. dressings) which the NP may have done themselves in the slightly longer consultation time allotted. The Centre for Innovation in Primary Care (2000) also observed that the time spent with patients was similar for PNs and GPs, but that nurses spent the extra time between consultations completing the necessary administration, which GPs would tend to do during the consultation. They suggest that this might lead to nurses giving the patient their more complete attention during the consultation, and hence to some of the better patient satisfaction outcomes.

One small study set in secondary care examined nurse-led follow-up of lung cancer patients, and traditional medical follow-up (Moore et al. 2002). Again, while both groups were satisfied with the care they received, those followed up by nurses were more satisfied and scored significantly higher in each subset measured. However, the model of follow-up adopted by the nurses was entirely different to that followed by the medical staff and resulted in far more time spent in contact with the patient, either by phone or face-to-face. It was a very supportive model of follow-up, addressing a wider, more holistic agenda than conventional medical follow-up. This would suggest that it may not only be the extra time spent in nurse consultations which is of value to the patient, it is how the nurse uses that the time and the model of care followed.

Diagnosis

Traditionally, diagnosis has been seen as the prerogative of the medical practitioner, with nurse involvement being informal and often unacknowledged (Baird 2001; Walby and Greenwall

1994). However, the DoH's (2006, section 7) working definition of independent prescribing is 'prescribing by a practitioner responsible and accountable for the assessment of patients with diagnosed and undiagnosed conditions, and for decisions about the clinical management required, including prescribing', which would suggest that diagnosis is now an accepted part of the role of all independent prescribers. Within the context of supplementary prescribing, it is expected that the independent prescribing partner would be responsible for the initial diagnosis and management plan. However, nurses working as supplementary prescribers would be experts within their fields of practice and would be expected to raise their concerns with the independent prescriber if they suspected an incorrect diagnosis. Interestingly, physiotherapists, who have long followed a medical model of problem solving and diagnosis are not, at the time of writing, able to qualify and practice as independent prescribers.

It has been suggested (Baird 2000a; 2000b) that nurses have for a long time been involved in the diagnosis of both acute and chronic disease, with many doctors openly acknowledging and accepting this. However, nurses are wise to remember that their initial training does not equip them for such a role. Similarly, pharmacists are familiar with consulting and reaching a decision about appropriate medication or advice in their role in the community, but have had little or no formal training in diagnostics. Many courses of varying quality are being developed to meet this need, but nurses and pharmacists training as independent/supplementary prescribers should remember that the prescribing course is not in itself designed to teach the clinical skills necessary for diagnosis (DoH 2006, section 19). Practitioners must already be deemed competent in the areas in which they intend to prescribe before they access the course.

In reaching a working diagnosis, the practitioner will go through several stages of data collection and analysis. Bates (1995) discusses in some depth the process of clinical decision making and establishing a working diagnosis, while acknowledging that it is not always possible to reach a definite diagnosis. Tate (2003) suggests that particularly within primary care, it may well not always be possible or even desirable to make a firm clinical diagnosis in order to formulate a management plan. For example, the patient presenting with a sore throat may have an illness which is viral or bacterial in origin, but as the management and outcome are essentially the same, there is no real need to differentiate in the majority of cases.

In reality, there will often exist an element of uncertainty about a diagnosis. It has been suggested that nurses can find tolerating uncertainty difficult (Luker et al. 1998). Traditionally, nurse training has not prepared nurses for this, as the risk has been borne by the doctor who has decided on, and taken responsibility for, the treatment. Medical training, in contrast, prepares doctors to make decisions in the face of uncertainty (Fox 1979; RCGP 1996). This is something that prescribing nurses and other practitioners will need to learn to manage as they accept responsibility for their own prescribing decisions.

Consultations with pharmacists

The concept of a pharmacist undertaking a consultation with a patient is also relatively new, though many community pharmacists have been consulting with the public for many years, albeit in an informal and unrecognised manner. Lack of privacy and the need for a private consulting room have been identified as a potential barrier to community pharmacists offering more formal consultations (Bellingham 2002a). However, a number of pharmacies are already participating in pilot schemes which enable them to directly supply simple remedies to patients who do not pay for their prescriptions (Bellingham 2002b) and these schemes are likely to be expanded in the future.

Literature on pharmacists' consultation skills is sparse, but the recent interest in clinical medication review (DoH 2001) has led to an increase in the number of practice-based pharmacists consulting directly with patients about their medication. Petty et al. (2003) suggest that while such a role is acceptable to a large number of patients, some remain suspicious, and further research is needed into the views of patients and carers. Chen and Britten (2000), in their study of medication reviews, observed that pharmacists conducting such reviews did not seem to experience any significant difficulties in communicating with patients. Consultations were relatively long as compared with nurse or doctor consultations (between 15 and 90 minutes) and patients would seem to value being able to spend time with a pharmacist in an unhurried environment. While the style and process of consultation are not explored, patients in this study divulged many of their beliefs about their medication to the pharmacist, many of which they had not felt able to discuss with the prescribing doctor. Whether this is a feature of consulting with a different practitioner to the original prescriber, or is something which pharmacist prescribers would also be able to elicit, is unknown.

Many pharmacists have developed skills in concordance which they will be able to bring to their consultations. Concordance, suggest Weiss and Britten (2003), refers to a consultation process and sharing of power between the professional and the patient. It values the patient's experience of illness and medication as much as the professional's expert knowledge. It is possible that pharmacist prescribers who have already developed expertise in this area may achieve better outcomes in their prescribing practice.

Consultations with other practitioners

There would appear to be very little literature specifically relating to consultations with other practitioners. One small study by Collins et al. (2003) examined the communication styles of nurses, doctors and other HCPs (dieticians and speech and language therapists), and concluded that the consulting style of other HCPs was more like that of nurses than doctors. There is clearly room for more research in this area, as other HCPs take on roles, including prescribing, which have traditionally been the preserve of the medical profession.

Decision making and prescribing

Within the context of the consultation, the prescriber will be faced with a number of decisions, including the formulation of a diagnosis or management plan, and whether or not to prescribe (Luker et al. 1998). The literature describes two broad models of decision making, the analytical and the intuitive. The analytical model describes a logical process of decision making (Harbison 1991; Miers 1990; Pauker and Karriser 1987) often using a decision tree or algorithm. A limitation of this method is that it assumes that all relevant knowledge is available to the practitioner, something which is often not the case in practice.

The intuitive model has been extensively discussed by Benner (1984), who describes five stages from novice to expert practitioner. Benner (1984) suggests that the method of decision making depends upon which stage the nurse is at in his or her professional development. The novice relies very much on an analytical method of decision making, as he or she has no experience to guide his or her thinking, while the expert practitioner also draws on intuitive knowledge gained by experience. Hamm (1988), however, views the analytic and the intuitive models as ends of a continuum, and suggests that practitioners will tend more towards the analytic end of the continuum the more time and information are available. In reality, most clinical decision making is likely to involve both analytic and intuitive aspects.

Influences on prescribing

In deciding whether, or what, to prescribe, clinicians are likely to be influenced by a number of factors. It has been suggested (Denig and Bradley 1998) that these fall into three main categories: pressure from patients; pressure from other prescribers; and other influences. In many cases, it may well be that a prescription is not the most appropriate response, especially in primary care where symptoms may be attributable to 'illness' rather than 'disease' (Stewart and Roter 1989).

A number of studies have suggested that doctors frequently prescribe in response to pressure from patients, either real or perceived (Bradley 1992; Britten 1994; Virji and Britten 1991). It may be that some patients do expect to leave the consultation with a prescription, but this is by no means always the case and the desire for explanation and reassurance is often underestimated (Barry et al. 2000; Britten et al. 2000). Doctors prescribe in response to patients' health beliefs, to preserve the doctor/patient relationship and to end a difficult or lengthy consultation. Non-medical prescribers would be naïve to think that they will be immune from such pressures.

Pressure from other prescribers can also be a factor in deciding on a prescription. Precedents set by 'specialists', prescribing colleagues and possibly even oneself in a previous encounter with the patient may all influence the outcome of a consultation. The pharmaceutical industry will have new prescribers in its sights, and clinicians are likely to be influenced by all these sources. Trust policies on prescribing will seek to influence prescribers and there may on occasions be conflicts between these policies and what the practitioner believes to be in the best interests of the patient. External influences include local formularies, clinical guidelines, NICE guidelines, the national service frameworks and the media, which is increasingly seeking to influence patients more directly. Prescribers will have to negotiate a path through these varying influences.

Hall et al. (2003) observed that a number of factors influence community nurses' decisions to prescribe, with the need to promote patient concordance emerging as a key influence. Another factor, which may be more pertinent to community practitioner prescribers (previously district nurse/health visitor prescribers) than independent prescribers, would appear to be whether or not the patient is exempt from prescription charges. Many of the items available to community pratitioner prescribers can be bought, and some (though by no means all) nurses reported being heavily influenced by the patient's status in respect of prescription charges (Hall et al. 2003; Luker et al. 1998). Given that prescription charges have recently been abolished in some areas of the UK, it remains to be seen how this might influence a patient's decision to seek a prescription, and the practitioner's decision to prescribe.

Principles of good prescribing

The National Prescribing Centre (NPC 1999) has developed a series of 'signposts', known as the 'prescribing pyramid' (Figure 3.1) to assist prescribers in decision making. These seven principles break down the complex process of prescribing into a series of steps which, if considered, may help practitioners to prescribe appropriately.

- Consider the patient. Thorough consideration of the holistic needs of the patient, including medical and social history, can help in deciding whether or not medication is indicated. A drug history, including OTC and alternative therapies, should be included along with any drug allergies or sensitivities.

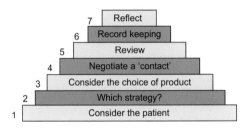

Figure 3.1 The prescribing pyramid (NPC 1999)

- Which strategy? Treatment options other than prescribing should always be considered, including explanation, reassurance and recommending the buying of OTC medication. The practitioner needs to discover and acknowledge the patient's expectations (Pendleton et al. 1984).
- Consider the choice of product. The NPC suggest the use of the mnemonic EASE to assist in deciding which product to prescribe, ie:

E – how **E**ffective is the product?

A – is it **A**ppropriate for this patient?

S – how **S**afe is it?

E – is the prescription cost-**E**ffective?

- Negotiate a contract. Prescribing should be viewed as shared decision making between the patient and the prescriber. Effective communication on the part of the prescriber is essential to ensure that the patient understands what the prescription is for, how long it takes to work, how to take it and how long for, what dose to take and any possible side effects.
- Review the patient. It is not good practice to issue repeat prescriptions without regular patient review, and the implementation guidelines for extended formulary nurse prescribers (DoH, 2002) suggest that nurses should not issue repeat prescriptions for more than six months without reassessment. However, this may lead to some tensions. For example, within general practice, many patients who are well established on the contraceptive pill are only reviewed annually. It would not be reasonable for the practice to have a different approach to those patients who initially saw the nurse. In reality, it is likely that those repeat prescriptions which were initiated by other prescrib-ers will be generated by receptionists along with prescriptions initiated by GPs, and will be signed by GPs. However, clinicians have a responsibility which goes beyond the initial prescribing decision, and should ensure that they are involved in practice discussions on repeat prescribing policy and medicines management.
- Keep records. The NMC guidelines on record keeping outline the standards expected of all nurses, and there are additional requirements for nurse prescribers to record their prescription in the GP records within 48 hours. Similar standards are expected of pharmacist prescribers (DoH 2002). Local policy as to how this is to be achieved will vary.
- Reflect. Reflecting on prescribing decisions, both alone and with colleagues, (possibly within the context of clinical supervision), will help practitioners to improve and develop their prescribing practice.

Computer decision support

With the proliferation of information technology in healthcare, the interest in computerised support has increased. A number of systems to assist in the process of decision making and prescribing have been developed, including Clinical Knowledge Summaries (cks.library.nhs. uk), which is well known in general practice; ISABEL (www.isabel.org.uk), a tool to support differential diagnosis in paediatric practice; and the Clinical Assessment System, used by NHS Direct. Given the ever-increasing scope of medical knowledge, and the vast number of potential treatments, there is no doubt that these systems should be able to facilitate better decision making, though how best to integrate them in the consultation remains a challenge (Eccles et al. 2002). There is a suggestion that those systems which interrupt the consultation with prompts are less well received by practitioners that those which can be accessed 'on demand' (Rousseau et al. 2003). It has also been suggested (Sullivan and Mitchell 1995) that using a computer within the consultation can tend to increase the doctor-initiated, 'medical' content of the consultation, at the expense of patient-initiated and 'social' content, while increasing the length of the consultation. However, there is no doubt that computers are here to stay, and used appropriately, they may have the potential to improve clinician performance (Sullivan and Mitchell 1995).

Conclusion

Nurses, pharmacists and other practitioners have sought the ability to prescribe for many years. It brings with it a new level of responsibility and accountability, and has the potential to alter the dynamics of the practitioner/patient relationship. Skills in communication and decision making are central to this relationship, whether or not the practitioner is a prescriber. Those new to prescribing may need to ensure that the ability to issue a prescription does not detract from other, equally important aspects of their relationship with the patient.

References

Baird, A. (2000a). Crown II: the implications of nurse prescribing for practice nurses. *British Journal of Community Nursing* 5(9): 454–461.

Baird, A. (2000b). Prescribing decisions in general practice. *Practice Nursing* 11(7): 9–12.

Baird, A. (2001). Diagnosis and prescribing. *Primary Health Care* 11(5): 24–26.

Barry, C.A., Bradley, C.P., Britten, N. et al. (2000). Patients' unvoiced agendas in general practice consultations. *British Medical Journal* 320: 1246–1250.

Bates, B. (1995). *A Guide to Physical Examination and History Taking* (sixth edition). Philadelphia, PA: JB Lippincott Company.

Bellingham, C. (2002a). Space, time and team working: issues for pharmacists who wish to prescribe. *The Pharmaceutical Journal* 268: 562–563.

Bellingham, C. (2002b). Pharmacists who prescribe: the reality. *The Pharmaceutical Journal* 268: 238–239.

Benner, P. (1984) *From Novice to Expert. Excellence and Power in Clinical Nursing Practice.* Menlo Park, CA: Addison Wesley Publishing Company.

Bond, S., Beck, S., Cunningham, F. et al. (1999). Testing a rating scale of video-taped consultations to assess performance of trainee nurse practitioners in general practice. *Journal of Advanced Nursing* 30(5): 1064–1072.

Bradley, C.P. (1992). Uncomfortable prescribing decisions: a critical incident study. *British Medical Journal* 304: 294–296.

Britten, N. (1994). Patient demand for prescriptions. A view from the other side. *Family Practice* 11: 62–66.

Britten, N., Stevenson, F., Barry, A. et al. (2000). Misunderstandings in prescribing decisions in general practice: a qualitative study. *British Medical Journal* 320: 484–488.

Byrne, P.S., Long, B.E.L. (1976). *Doctors talking to patients*. London: HMSO.

The Centre for Innovation in Primary Care (2000). *What Do Practice Nurses Do? A Study of Roles, Responsibilities and Patterns of Work*. Sheffield: The Centre for Innovation in Primary Care.

Chant, S., Jenkinson, T., Randle, J. et al. (2002). Communication skills: some problems in nurse education and practice. *Journal of Clinical Nursing* 11(1): 12–21.

Chen, J., Britten, N. (2000). 'String medicine': an analysis of pharmacist consultations in primary care. *Family Practice* 17(6): 480–483.

Collins, S., Watt, I., Drew, P. et al. (2003). *Effective Consultations with Patients: a Comparative Multidisciplinary Study*. York: University of York.

Denig, P., Bradley, C. (1998). How doctors choose drugs. In: Hobbs, R., Bradley, C. *Prescribing in Primary Care*. Oxford: Oxford Medical Publications.

Department of Health (2001). *Medicines and Older People: Implementing Medicines Related Aspects of the National Service Framework for Older People*. London: DoH.

Department of Health (2002). *Extending Independent Nurse Prescribing Within the NHS in England*. London: DoH.

Department of Health (2006). *Improving Access to Medicines: a Guide to Implementing Nurse and Pharmacist Independent Prescribing within the NHS in England*. London: DoH.

Drucquer, M., Hutchinson, S. (2000). *The Consultation Toolkit. A Practical Method for Teaching and Learning Consultation Skills*. Sutton: Reed Healthcare Publishing.

Eccles, M., McColl, E., Steen, N. et al. (2002). Effect of computerised evidence based guidelines on management of asthma and angina in adults in primary care: cluster randomised controlled trial. *British Medical Journal* 325: 941–947.

Fox, R. (1979). *Essays in Medical Sociology*. New York, NY: John Wiley and Sons.

Greco, M., Powell, R. (2002). A patient feedback tool. *Primary Health Care* 12(10): 38–41.

Hall, J., Cantrill, J., Noyce, P. (2003). Influences on community nurse prescribing. *Nurse Prescribing* 1(3): 127–132.

Hamm, R.M. (1988). Clinical intuition and clinical analysis: expertise and the cognitive continuum. In: Dowie, J., Elstein, A. (eds.) *Professional Judgement – A Reader In Clinical Decision Making*. Cambridge: Cambridge University Press.

Harbison, J. (1991). Clinical decision making in nursing. *Journal of Advanced Nursing* 16: 404–407.

Hastings, A., Redsell, S. (2006). *The Good Consultation Guide for Nurses*. Oxford: Radcliffe Publishing.

Horrocks, S., Anderson, E., Salisbury, C. (2002). Systematic review of whether nurse practitioners working in primary care can provide equivalent care to doctors. *British Medical Journal* 324: 819–823.

Kemm, J., Close, A. (1995). *Health Promotion Theory and Practice*. London: Macmillan Press Ltd.

Kinnersley, P., Anderson, E., Parry, K. et al. (2000). Randomised controlled trial of nurse practitioner versus general practitioner care for patients requesting 'same day' consultations in primary care. *British Medical Journal* 320: 1043.

Launer, J. (2002). *Narrative Based Primary Care. A Practical Guide*. Oxford: Radcliffe Medical Press.

Luker, K., Hogg, C., Austin, L. et al. (1998). Decision making: the context of nurse prescribing. *Journal of Advanced Nursing* 27: 657–665.

Maguire, P., Pitceathly, C. (2002). Key communication skills and how to acquire them. *British Medical Journal* 325: 697–700.

Miers, M. (1990). Developing skills in decision making. *Nursing Times* 86(30): 32–33.

Moore, S., Corner, J., Haviland, J. et al. (2002). Nurse led follow up and conventional medical follow up in management of patients with lung cancer: randomised trial. *British Medical Journal* 325: 1145–1147.

National Prescribing Centre (1999). Nurse prescribing bulletin. Signposts for prescribing nurses – general principles of good prescribing. http://www.npc.co.uk/prescribers/resources/nurse_bulletin_vol1no1.pdf

Neighbour, R. (1987). *The inner consultation: how to develop an effective and intuitive consulting style.* Lancaster: MTP Press.

Pauker, S.G., Karriser, J.P. (1987). Medical progress decision analysis. *New England Journal of Medicine 316*(5): 250–258.

Pendleton, D., Schofield, T., Tate, P. et al. (1984). *The consultation: an approach to learning and teaching.* Oxford: Oxford University Press.

Petty, D.R., Knapp, P., Raynor, D.K. et al. (2003). Patients' views of a pharmacist-run medication review clinic in general practice. *British Journal of General Practice 53*: 607–613.

Reveley, S. (1998). The role of the triage nurse practitioner in general medical practice: an analysis of the role. *Journal of Advanced Nursing 28*(3): 584–591.

Rosenstock, I.M. (1974). The health belief model and preventative health behaviour. In: Becker, M. (ed.) *The Health Belief Model and Personal Health Behaviour.* Thorafore, NJ: Charles Slack.

Rotter, J.B. (1954). *Social Learning and Clinical Psychology.* Englewood Cliffs, NJ: Prentice-Hall.

Rousseau, N., McColl, E., Newton, J. et al. (2003). Practice based, longitudinal, qualitative interview study of computerised evidence based guidelines in primary care. *British Medical Journal 326*: 314–322.

Royal College of General Practitioners (1996). *The Nature of General Medical Practice.* London: RCGP.

Shum, C., Humphreys, A., Wheeler, D. et al. (2000). Nurse management of patients with minor illness in general practice: multicentre, randomised controlled trial. *British Medical Journal 320*: 1038–1043.

Silverman, J., Kurtz, S., Draper, J. (1998). *Skills for Communicating with Patients.* Oxford: Radcliffe Medical Press.

Stewart, M.A., Roter, D. (eds.) (1989). *Communicating with Medical Patients.* Newbury Park: Sage.

Stott, N.C.H., Davies, R.H. (1979). The exceptional potential in each primary care consultation. *Journal of the Royal College of General Practitioners 29*: 210–215.

Sullivan, F., Mitchell, E. (1995). Has general practitioner computing made a difference to patient care? A systematic review of published reports. *British Medical Journal 311*: 848–852.

Tate, P. (2003). *The Doctor's Communication Handbook* (4th edition). Oxford: Radcliffe Medical Press.

Virji, A., Britten, N. (1991). A study of the relationship between patients' attitudes and doctors' prescribing. *Family Practice 8*: 314–319.

Walby S., Greenwall, J. (1994). Medicine and Nursing: Professions in a Changing Health Service. London: Sage.

Weiss, M., Britten, N. (2003). What is concordance? *The Pharmaceutical Journal 271*(7270): 493.

While, A. (2002). Practical skills: prescribing consultation in practice. *British Journal of Community Nursing, 7*(9): 469–473.

Legal aspects of independent and supplementary prescribing

Mark Gagan

This chapter sets out to give a precise account of the history of changes brought about by the desire to change prescribing authority, and give definitions of independent and supplementary prescribing, patient group directions (PGDs) and their possible implications for non-medical prescribers (NMPs).

There is a short introduction to how the law is formulated, the differences between civil and criminal law, and how issues such as duty of care, negligence, consent and accountability might affect interactions with patients. Professional issues, such as teamwork and communication, are also addressed. Cases that have gone before the courts are highlighted in an attempt to illustrate how the law has been previously applied. The role of regulatory bodies, such as the Nursing and Midwifery Council and the Health Professions Council, are also noted throughout.

It appears that legal issues are a constant source of worry and fascination for many healthcare practitioners. During the years 2007–2008 some 5400 claims of clinical negligence and 3380 claims of non-clinical negligence were received by the National Health Service Litigation Authority (NHSLA). This resulted in a cost of £633 million paid out in clinical negligence claims (NHSLA 2009). The National Patient Safety Agency report, *Safety in Doses: Medication Safety Incidents in the NHS* (NPSA 2007), indicates that over 736 million items were prescribed in England, at a cost of £8 billion, in 2006. The scale of activity is enormous. Alongside this, the potential for medication error is substantial throughout the whole medication management process – assessment, prescribing, preparing, dispensing and administering the drugs appropriately and safely.

In 2006, nurses prescribed almost 5.5 million items, with pharmacists accounting for 23 000 prescribable items (NPSA 2007). This is in response to Governmental policies designed to provide easier, speedy access to NHS services for the general public (particularly those who are seen to be in socially disadvantaged groups and traditionally therefore less able to access primary care facilities easily).

Legislation relevant to prescribing

The Medicines Act 1968 regulates the licensing, supply and administration of medicines.

The Act also requires the Secretary of State for Health to place on the prescription only list medicines that represent a danger to patients if their use is not supervised by an appropriate practitioner (Medicines Act 1968 s58 (2) (b), cited in Griffith 2006).

The Act also regulates medicines into three categories:

- Prescription Only Medicines (POMs). These are medicines which may be supplied or administered on the instruction of an appropriate practitioner (doctor or dentist), and certain approved medications from nurse prescribers and allied healthcare practitioners, such as pharmacists, podiatrists and optometrists.

- Pharmacy Only Medications (P). These can be purchased from a registered primary care pharmacy provided a pharmacist supervises the sale.
- General Sales List (GSL). These require neither a prescription nor supervision from a pharmacist, usually being available from retail outlets.

The Act also states that:

- An appropriate practitioner is: 'a doctor, dentist or veterinary surgeon'.
- A specific prescription is always required for the supply of a POM.
- A prescription for a POM has to come from 'an appropriate practitioner'.

A POM can be administered by a 'doctor, dentist or veterinary surgeon' or 'a person acting on the instruction of an appropriate practitioner' (Pennels 1999).

This means that only those who are stated to be 'appropriate practitioners' can prescribe POMs.

The Cumberlege report (DHSS 1986) concluded that community nurses should be given access to prescribing rights. This was followed by the first Crown report (DoH 1989), which argued that community nurses and health visitors should be able to prescribe from a 'nurses' formulary' – limited in number but useful enough to enable measurable time saving and cost benefits for patients, general practitioners and community nurses.

The Medicinal Products: Prescriptions by Nurses etc Act (1992), which amended the National Health Service Act 1997 (s41) and the Medicines Act 1968 (s58), and the Medicinal Products: Prescriptions by Nurses etc Act 1992 (Commencement No 1) Order 1994, enabled those nurses on Parts 1 and 12 (registered general nurses) of the United Kingdom Central Council (UKCC) register, who also possessed a district nurse qualification or who were on Part 11 (health visitors) and who had undergone further training, to prescribe products from a limited list known as the Nurse Prescribers' Formulary (NPF) (Pennels 1999).

The success of nurse prescribing encouraged legislators to further the cause. The Pharmaceutical Services Regulations (1994) allowed pharmacists to legally accept and dispense prescriptions written by nurses (Gibson 2001). The second Crown report (*Review of Prescribing, Supply and Administration of Medicines*, DoH 1999) proposed the introduction of a new framework of prescribing, supply and administration of medicines whereby the majority of patients would receive medicines on an individual patient-specific basis, the prescribing authority of doctors, dentists, district nurses and health visitors would continue and that this prescribing authority would be extended to include new groups of healthcare professionals.

The trend continued with the Health and Social Care Act 2001 (s63) when the Government extended prescribing rights to pharmacists and introduced the concept of extended formulary nurse prescribers and supplementary prescribers.

In 2000, PGDs were introduced to try to clear the legal ambiguity of nurses giving medication, agreed by medical staff under the umbrella term of 'administration via protocol'. PGDs are defined as 'a written instruction for the supply and administration of medicines to groups of patients who may not be individually identified before presenting for treatment' (NMC 2006).

PGDs are not a form of prescribing and there is no specific training that health professionals must undertake before supplying or administering medicines in this way (DoH 2003a). Further guidance is available in Health Service Circular 2000/026 and in Home Office Circular 049/2003 *Controlled Drugs Legislation – Nurse Prescribing and Patient Group Directions*.

In July 2005 the Nursing and Midwifery Council confirmed that following amendments to the definitions of District Nurse/Health Visitor Prescriber and Extended Formulary Prescriber by the Health Care and Associated Professions Orders 2004/1756 and 2004/1771, any first level nurse could access training to become a nurse prescriber. There are of course several caveats regarding specialist knowledge, competence and skills before any first level nurse can enter training as a nurse prescriber (NMC 2005).

Definitions of independent and supplementary prescriber

'Independent prescribing' is prescribing by a practitioner (doctor, dentist, nurse or pharmacist) responsible and accountable for the assessment of patients with undiagnosed or diagnosed conditions and for decisions about the clinical management required, including prescribing. Within medicines legislation, the term used is 'appropriate practitioner' and 'in partnership with the patient . . . it requires an initial patient assessment, interpretation of that assessment, a decision on safe and appropriate therapy and a process for ongoing monitoring. The independent prescriber is responsible and accountable for at least this element of the patient's care' (DoH 2006). The Medicines and Human Use (Prescribing) (Miscellaneous Amendments) Order 2006 and associated medicine regulation amendments enabled those nurses who had completed a nurse independent prescribing course to prescribe any licensed medicine, including some controlled drugs, for any medical condition within their clinical competence. A similar notion of independent prescribing for pharmacists was introduced, with the significant difference that these independent pharmacist prescribers will not be able to prescribe any controlled drugs although community pharmacists can sell Schedule 5 controlled drugs. (DoH 2006).

Supplementary prescribing is defined as 'a voluntary partnership between an independent prescriber who for the purposes of supplementary prescribing must be a doctor or a dentist and a supplementary prescriber to implement an agreed patient specific Clinical Management Plan (CMP) with the patient's agreement' (DoH 2003b).

Nurse, pharmacist and allied health professional supplementary prescribers are able to prescribe any medicine, including controlled drugs and unlicensed medicines that are listed in the agreed CMP for any medical condition, provided they do so under the terms of a patient-specific CMP agreed with a doctor (DoH 2006).

The legal system in England and Wales

Essentially there are two branches of law; civil and criminal.

Civil law usually deals with disputes where one person who may have suffered loss or harm (the claimant) brings a legal action against another person (the defendant) who the claimant believes has caused them loss or harm. This may be referred to as a 'tort' or civil wrong, which could include negligence or assault (due to a lack of consent). If the claim is proven then the defendant may be liable for damages and have to pay monetary compensation to ameliorate the situation as far as is possible.

Criminal law involves offences against the State (the law of the land rather than private individuals) and it is usually the Crown that brings the action against the defendant.

There is also a system of courts, civil and criminal, that deal with all actions in law.

In civil courts all evidence is presented before a judge who makes a decision on the evidence presented before the court. In criminal cases, most start at the magistrates' court and move upwards in court hierarchy, depending on the severity of the alleged offence. In some cases evidence may be presented to a judge and jury and it is in these cases that the jury, based on the evidence placed before them, decide whether the defendant is guilty or not guilty of the alleged offence.

Sources of law

The law of the land is primarily made using two devices.

Statute law

Statutes are Acts of Parliament, which are presented via the House of Commons following a long established process that involves debate and argument before being moved on to the House of Lords. Here further debate takes place and requests for changes (amendments) are usually made before the Bill (as the statutes are called before being finally agreed) is returned to the House of Commons for final discussion. On completion of these debates the Bill is given Royal Assent (the approval and signing of the Bill by the reigning Monarch) and passes into law.

Common law (sometimes known as judge-made law)

In cases where there is no existing Act of Parliament to cover a particular occurrence, the legal system looks for similar cases that have been decided in the past by judges.

There is a legal term known as 'precedent', which indicates that cases showing similar facts and similar progressions to previous cases should be dealt with in a 'like for like' manner. This system works on the premise that the higher the court making the decision is in the legal system, the more binding its decisions are on the courts below it. The highest court under the England and Wales system was traditionally the House of Lords, with its decisions expected to be followed by every junior court below it. In October 2009, the House of Lords was replaced by the Supreme Court as the primary court of the judiciary. However, there is the possibility that certain cases can go before the European Court of Law, as the United Kingdom is a member of the European Union and subject, in certain circumstances, to European law, which may trump the decisions of the House of Lords. The fact that judges act in a certain manner has implications for non-medical prescribers, particularly where cases of negligence or duty of care standards are being considered.

Negligence

For negligence to be proven, the claimant has to meet the following criteria:

(a) a duty of care is owed by the defendant (a non-medical prescriber, for example) to the claimant, and

(b) the defendant breached that duty by failing to exercise reasonable care, and

(c) the breach of duty caused the claimant's injuries and those injuries are reasonably foreseeable as a result of that breach of duty.

In essence, the onus is therefore on the claimant to prove on the balance of probability that the defendant's acts or omissions left them in a worse state than before they had been treated by the defendant. If the claimant fails in any one of the three criteria to prove that the defendant was culpable then the case against the defendant will not succeed and the claimant will not be entitled to any recompense. The standard of proof in civil cases is less than that in criminal cases where it must be 'proven beyond reasonable doubt' that the person is guilty of a particular act.

Duty of care

The claimant has to prove on the balance of probabilities that the defendant owed them a duty of care. The legal precedent for establishing duty of care can be exemplified in Donoghue v

Stevenson [1932] AC 562 where a manufacturer was held liable for the injuries received by the claimant who had consumed a bottle of ginger beer that contained the remains of a dead snail and as a result had developed gastroenteritis. The case produced the 'neighbour principle' which states that a duty of care is owed to anyone who is reasonably likely to be affected by one's acts and omissions (Hendrick 2000). Although it may appear unlikely that a bottle of ginger beer containing snail remains has anything to do with a practitioner's daily work, it must be remembered that precedent can apply across a whole series of circumstances even though at first sight, there appears to be little in common between cases.

Once a duty of care has been established, it has to be shown that the practitioner failed to honour that commitment and caused a breach of that duty to occur. The practitioner's actions would have to be examined to see if they reached the accepted level of competence.

The legal standard of care is classically defined in the case of Bolam v Friern Hospital Management Committee [1957] WLR 582. This case is important because it stated the famous legal dictum '...a doctor is not guilty of negligence, if he has acted in accordance with a practice accepted as proper by a responsible body of medical men skilled in that particular art'.

The language may seem archaic now but the implication is crucial. It may not be 'medical men' that are judged; it could be nurses, pharmacists, midwives or community practitioners. The names are not important – it is the job being done that is under scrutiny. This is an important benchmark for practitioners as it implies that they will be judged against the standard of their peers. The courts might set up the test but it is up to the professionals to decide whether or not the test has been passed. This may seem to favour the practitioner rather than the claimant and has been a source of debate over many years. This situation has been questioned by senior judges, who appear to indicate a degree of scepticism might be useful when considering the evidence of expert peers.

The idea that 'doctor knows best' is no longer considered a 'copper bottomed guarantee' of certainty, particularly following the Bolitho case. This concerned the treatment of a young child, who, it was claimed, suffered injury through the allegedly negligent behaviour of a doctor who did not attend him when requested to do so. The child's condition was extremely serious and it was argued that it was highly unlikely that the child would have survived unscathed even if the doctor concerned had intubated him.

Expert opinion at the time of the trial indicated this to be the likely outcome. However, the judge was not so convinced of the rationale supplied by the experts and said that greater emphasis should be placed on logical and defensible evidence-based practice (see later discussion).

The final stage in the process of proving negligence is to examine if the damage or injury occurred as a result of the practitioner's actions.

If it were to be shown that the actions (or omissions) taken by the practitioner were inappropriate and it could be reasonably foreseen that damage or injury would occur as a result of the practitioner's actions, then it could be stated that the charge of negligence would be well founded. The practitioner would therefore be liable for damages (fiscal compensation and possibly the legal costs of both parties) and may face the possibility of disciplinary action from their employer also.

The legal situation may be less problematic in some cases. For instance, a charge of negligence may not be upheld by the court, so no legal liability would exist for the practitioner, however, the professional standard of care might interest the regulatory bodies (NMC, HPC, RPSGB), who might wish to examine the professional competence of their registrant. So although the practitioner may not have committed a criminal offence or civil offence, the regulatory authority might consider that the profession has been brought into disrepute as a result of the practitioner's actions and, as a result, might consider applying sanctions (including removal from the register), which can have dire effects on the practitioner's ability to remain in employment.

In a recent case involving the dispensing of beta blockers, rather than the prescribed prednisolone tablets, a pharmacist faced a potential prison sentence if found guilty of causing the death of a patient who had taken the incorrectly labelled medication. The medical evidence indicated the woman had died as a result of natural causes. The pharmacist was found not guilty of the death of the woman, however, following the case, the pharmacist resigned from the RPSGB and as a result is no longer able to practice as a pharmacist.

A second example involves the removal from the nursing register of a nurse prescriber who prescribed sildenafil for her husband. She also altered his computer records and did not check any incompatibilities with his current medication (which were present). This was in violation of several ethical and legal precepts as well as breaching much of the NMC's code of practice (NMC 2008). She was removed from the nursing register as a result.

Teamwork

In supplementary prescribing the interaction between the IP (doctor or dentist) and the SP is maintained on a voluntary basis. The working relationship is expected to be a close one between the professionals and it should be noted 'good prescribing practice requires the patient is considered an equal partner to ensure informed consent' (the Task Force on Medicines Partnership 2002, cited in NPC 2003). Most legal authorities would encourage openness and sharing as it indicates a willingness to engage patients in a transparent manner (see Consent, below).

Responsibilities

Prescribing partners must work together in an open, co-operative manner that ensures lawful supplementary prescribing. This means that:

- The IP is a doctor or dentist.
- The SP is a registered nurse, registered midwife, registered pharmacist or other AHP able to use this route.
- A written CMP exists relating to a named patient and to that patient's specific conditions. Agreement to the plan must be recorded by both the IP and the SP before supplementary prescribing begins.
- The IP and the SP share, consult, have access to and use the same patient record (NPC 2003).

These aspirations are echoed in the NMC code (NMC 2008), which states:

'You must work cooperatively within teams and respect the skills, expertise and contributions of your colleagues' and 'you must consult and take advice from colleagues when appropriate' as well as 'you must make a referral to another practitioner when it is in the best interests of someone in your care'. Of course, not all prescribers are nurses; the exhortation is one aspiring to the use of best practice, which is something all practitioners should be working towards.

If a situation arose where a charge of negligence was brought that involved a supplementary practitioner, a defence of 'team' rather than 'individual responsibility' for the error would not be a valid defence. In law, there is no such thing as 'team liability'.

This was shown in the case of Prendergast v Sam Dee [1989] Med LR 36 where a doctor prescribed Amoxil but his writing was so illegible, the pharmacist thought Daonil had been prescribed and dispensed this to the patient instead. Unfortunately, the patient took the medication and became permanently brain damaged as a result of the error. The court found in favour of the claimant and awarded over £139 000. The doctor was found 25% liable (so had to pay 25% of the sum concerned) while the pharmacist paid the remaining 75%. Best practice would suggest that each practitioner is personally and professionally accountable for their own actions performed in the course of their work. The NMC code (NMC 2008) states:

'As a professional, you are personally accountable for your actions and omissions in your practice and must always be able to justify your decisions.'

This underlines the importance of being able to defend decisions made in the course of practice. Research-based care delivered promptly and appropriately is becoming the 'gold standard' approach to patient care delivery.

In the case of Bolitho v City and Hackney Health Authority [1997] 4 All ER 771 HL, a young child suffered brain damage following a cardiac arrest. One of the main issues was whether the doctor's failure to intubate the child (who had previously, that same afternoon, suffered two apparent airway occlusions) actually contributed to the cardiac arrest. If the failure to intubate was deemed to be unreasonable behaviour, would this mean the doctor would have fallen short of their duty of care to the child?

It was found that there was a reasonable body of expert opinion that stated it might be considered reasonable not to intubate the child and as such, the doctor was not liable under the Bolam test.

Since this case, judges have been much more reticent to accept expert opinion, just on the face of it. There has to be logical and credible evidence to support the expert opinion.

In 2001 Lord Woolf, then Chief Justice, stated the phrase 'doctor knows best' (perhaps with the Bolam test in mind) might better be rephrased as 'doctor knows best if he acts reasonably and logically and gets his facts right' (www.maxfac.com 2001). This was a real challenge to the notion that practitioners (and by implication they are the experts) know best and that this is sufficient reason to believe what they say. It is a call to all practitioners to be fully accountable and in doing so be able to defend their care or their acts and omissions on a sound basis that stands up to robust examination. The NMC code (NMC 2008) is quite clear about this: 'You must deliver care on the best available evidence or best practice' and 'you must have the knowledge and skills for safe and effective practice when working without direct supervision'.

There are obvious implications for lifelong learning and the application of evidence-based research into daily practice here. A practitioner's knowledge cannot remain static because care itself is dynamic with new treatments and procedures being introduced on an almost daily basis. The law requires practitioners to demonstrate an awareness of new methods of practice. This is demonstrated in the case of Gascoigne v Ian Sheridan and Co and Latham [1994] 5 Med LR 437, cited in Hendrick (2000), where a consultant was questioned on his responsibility to keep up-to-date with changes in techniques that affected his particular field of expertise. The judge in the case agreed that professionals had a duty to be aware of mainstream changes but need not be cognisant of every change that occurred as this would prove to be time consuming and difficult to maintain.

In the field of non-medical prescribing where policy initiatives, legal changes and new drugs appear at a dramatic rate, it would be impractical to be aware of every development as it happened, however, refreshing one's knowledge and practice regularly will be an expectation of employers and the general public. This is particularly pertinent if a practitioner prescribes a product that, by virtue of its manufacture or because of inappropriate administration or poor instruction, causes damage to a patient.

The Consumer Protection Act 1987

This Act can be utilised to bring a claim where a defective product has caused harm. This is defined as 'there is a defect in a product…if the safety of the product is not such as persons generally are entitled to expect' (Consumer Protection Act 1987, cited in Dimond 2002). The claimant does not have to prove the defendant was negligent, rather that the prescriber used a defective product. The outcome of this legislation is that a prescriber who gives a dressing or medication to a patient that is found to be defective in some way and causes the patient harm, is potentially liable as the supplier of a defective product under the Act. The supplier could therefore be an independent (doctor, nurse or pharmacist) or supplementary prescriber (nurse or pharmacist). This has implications for understanding the supply mechanisms within the organisation for which one works and using a system where checks can be made that would enable a product to be traced back to its original source (the supplier).

The practitioner in all cases must be knowledgeable about the product supplied and be aware of any problems associated with its use. Prompt and precise recording of any actual or potential problems encountered in use would be desirable, along with the circumstances of their occurrence. Careful checking of information on how to use the particular product, its storage, disposal and anticipated side effects, and recording of what had been said and shown to the patient with regard to the product, would indicate that reasonable care had been take to inform the patient, should a case come to litigation.

The practitioner is also responsible for notifying the appropriate authorities regarding any adverse drug reactions or defective medical devices. The Medicines and Healthcare Regulatory Authority (MHRA) and the Commission on Human Medicines (CHM) are responsible for the safety of medicines and medical devices and for the prompt notification or withdrawal of any products that are found to be defective. The most well-known scheme is the 'Yellow Card' system of notifying adverse drug reactions, where anyone who has suffered an untoward reaction can notify the authorities immediately. This system hopes to improve the quality and effectiveness of medicinal products by highlighting dangers quickly, so that steps can be taken to enhance patient safety.

Consent

The expectations of the courts and regulatory bodies regarding consent are particularly demanding. There are several important cases that have helped shape the ways courts have dealt with practitioners who have acted without consent. One such case is Scholendorff v Society of New York Hospital [1914] 105 NE 92, in which Judge Cardozo established that each adult person, of sound mind, has the right to accept or refuse medical treatment (including the taking of prescribed medication). To force treatment upon them (unless allowed by a court order) is to commit the offence of trespass (even assault or battery) to that person. This can lead to prosecution of the practitioner in a court of law.

Although this case is an example of American law, because the legal systems used by the United States and England and Wales are so similar, occasionally these judgements are used to inform and support judgements made in English and Welsh law. The 'Cardozo judgement' is one such example. All healthcare regulatory bodies insist their registrants seek the informed consent of patients involved before they engage in any treatment, thereby protecting themselves from any allegations of malpractice. The NMC code (NMC 2008) states: 'You must ensure that you gain consent before you begin any treatment or care' and 'you must respect and support people's rights to accept or decline treatment and care'.

Practitioners must be aware that when gaining consent, it must be valid, informed consent – without this, any consent gained may be termed invalid and therefore not recognised in law. Consent, when given, must be voluntary, made by a legally competent person, who is able to understand and retain the information given, therefore making an informed choice about their treatment. The person may also refuse treatment, even if this appears to fly in the face of logic or reason (as far as the practitioner is concerned).

This right was supported in Re C (adult – refusal of medical treatment) [1994] 1 All ER 819. The case concerned a patient (C) incarcerated in a special hospital who had developed gangrene in his foot, which if untreated, the medical staff agreed, would probably kill him. The recommended treatment was amputation of the diseased part. C refused to undergo the procedure and took his case to court where it was established that despite his illness, he understood the reason why an operation was deemed necessary and the likely consequences of his refusal to consent to the amputation.

The court found in his favour and declared him legally competent to refuse the operation despite the concerns of the healthcare staff caring for him. This can be distressing for the staff but the autonomy of the patient must be respected.

This case highlights the importance of open, honest communication between the practitioner and the patient. It should also encourage practitioners to be dutiful in their assessment of a patient's understanding of procedures or treatments that might be prescribed for them and to carefully record the interactions and information given.

The patient has a right to expect honest, truthful information and a right to request further clarification and a second opinion if they wish to seek one.

The question of how much information needs to be given is an important one. A simple answer might be along the lines that the amount of information given must be enough to enable the patient to make an informed choice about the risks for and against the course of treatment prescribed.

Once this information has been given and considered, and the patient has made the decision to freely give their consent to treatment, the practitioner cannot be accused of acting without consent. The use of concise factual, contemporaneous written records, indicating what information had been discussed and agreed upon by the patient and practitioner, would also be a useful safeguard in the case of confusion or if a dispute arose at a later date.

Such a case arose in McLennan v Newcastle Health Authority [1992] Med LR 215 where the claimant argued she had not been advised of the potential risks of her operation.

The defendant surgeon produced notes written at the time that indicated that the patient was told of the potential risks and that she had understood the implications of undergoing the planned surgery. The court found in favour of the surgeon on the basis of the entries in the patient's notes and the claimant lost the case.

Another case underlines the importance of explanation regarding the risks of treatment. In Chester v Afshar [2004] UK HL 41 [2004] 3 WLR 927, the claimant suffered from lower back pain and consulted Mr Afshar, a renowned consultant neurosurgeon. In the course of the discussion the surgeon outlined the expected outcomes of the case (Miss Chester was to have three intervertebral discs removed) and mentioned that there was a 1–2% chance of a condition that might cause 'cauda equine syndrome' (leading to paralysis and loss of function in the lower limbs). Although the claimant asked how likely this might be, the surgeon allegedly replied: 'Well I haven't paralysed anyone yet'. This remark was seen to be crucial in deciding the outcome of the case. The claimant later stated that had she been properly (and not, as she felt, flippantly) made aware of the dangers of cauda equine syndrome, she would have at least wanted a second opinion or the chance to talk things through at a later time prior to surgery. Despite her nervousness over the operation, Miss Chester agreed to the procedure. Unfortunately the risk eventuated and she was left with loss of both motor and sensory function below L2 level of her spinal column and paralysis. She took the case to court where it was decided the information given by the surgeon was not of an appropriate standard to enable her to make an informed decision. Once again, the importance of a proper assessment of the patient's understanding, ability to weigh up consequences and make an informed judgement regarding a prescribed course of treatment is vital. The fact that this information has been explained and that the patient states they understand the risks involved should be recorded contemporaneously and possibly signed by the patient in the patient record for greater clarification should the treatment ever have to be justified in court.

It has always been an established principle that no-one can consent to treatment for another adult. Hence, a wife cannot consent for a husband or a sister for a brother. If the person is unable to consent, say through unconsciousness due to a fall or head injury, then the practitioner must make a decision to start or withhold treatment in the patient's 'best interests'. These best interests may be informed by those who are closest to the patient, as they may be able to suggest what the patient may have wanted or definitely not wanted regarding medical intervention. However, it is the decision of the practitioner, not the next of kin, to act in the case of best interests.

There are occasions where the medical team and the next of kin cannot agree on the best way forward or there are massive ethical disagreements between relatives and practitioners. These cases might then be brought to the courts for the ultimate decision on the way forward.

It is not unknown for the courts to issue treatment orders against the specific wishes of patients using the rationale of best interests. The case of Re MB (adult – refusal of treatment) [1997] 2 FLR 426 CA showed how the courts can view an emergency situation and decide that certain factors (pain, fear of drugs) can render a patient 'incompetent' of making an informed decision regarding the acceptance or refusal of medical treatment and in those circumstances they can order treatment to be administered in the best interests of the patient. The case cited related to the delivery of a child by a caesarean operation. The mother had originally agreed to the procedure but withdrew her consent on realising she would have to have an anaesthetic administered by hypodermic injection. The mother had a 'needle phobia' and was adamant that she would not be injected at any time. The court ordered she should undergo the procedure and that staff could utilise any means necessary to undertake the operation without the mother's express permission. The child was delivered safely. The step was not taken lightly by the court, which emphasised the urgent nature of this situation, in this case overriding the wishes of the individual.

Since the passing of the Mental Capacity Act 2005, persons known as LPAs (Lasting Powers of Attorney) can make decisions regarding healthcare for patients who have previously signed that they wish a nominated LPA to make decisions about treatment for them, should the patient become incapable of making decisions for themselves at a later date. They cannot make end-of-life decisions (withdrawal of life support, etc.), however, everyday treatment issues will require their consent prior to treatment starting. Medical staff, where there are areas of dispute, may refer cases to the Court of Protection, which will make a final decision regarding treatment in the best interests of the incapacitated person.

More recent events

There has been much consternation recently regarding the issue of mixing medications within the same syringe, nebuliser or even hypodermic syringe. The practice has long been promoted without any problem. However, the Chartered Society of Physiotherapists (CSP) recently sought clarification of a potential issue whereby members of the CSP might find themselves in a quandary and facing potential illegal action by the mixing of medications in direct confrontation with the Medicine Act 1968.

The mixing of medications, where one medication was the vehicle for another to be administered, would be legal provided the substance was one recognised as a proper vehicle (i.e. sodium chloride 0.9% or water for injections). However, if the substance was neither of these two components, then the new compound produced by the two substances would be a new formula under the Medicine Act 1968 and therefore would be unlicensed (as a licence had not been granted for its manufacture). Administration would leave the practitioner, the CSP argued, open to potential criminal proceedings. Not only were physiotherapists exposed to this 'loophole' in the law, it meant care in the community, particularly in the area of palliative care, was also at risk of breaking the law because many drugs are administered via syringe drivers which invariably cause mixing of separate medications. The potential for disruption to everyday care was enormous.

The MHRA released a statement whereby it essentially pronounced that no prosecutions for the mixing of medications in palliative care would be instigated, unless it was in the public interest to prosecute certain cases that were obviously so inappropriate that they could not be ignored. Unfortunately, many common drug mixes, in daily use, were not in the palliative field and as the MHRA had only mentioned 'palliative care' as the exception to prosecution, many practitioners were still at risk of falling foul of the law. A consultation programme was announced (MLX 356) seeking interested parties' contributions on how to best solve the problem.

In July 2009, the MHRA issued further guidance to practitioners who mix medications as part of a well-established treatment regime, stating that those practitioners would not be prosecuted by the MHRA provided the care given was in the patient's best interests and consistent with established practice. Of course this was not a literal 'get out of jail free' card for those practitioners who might make errors or who might be negligent in their prescribing of medications. The MHRA stated they would look at any cases brought to their attention on a singular basis before deciding whether or not to take legal action. This statement, then, is essentially the same as for practitioners working in palliative care. There will be a review of the Medicines Act 1968 to enable this change to take place.

The opportunity to review the Medicines Act 1968, which is over 40 years old (and very much a creature of its time) means a new Act could incorporate all the changes to medicines and prescribing that were never envisaged at the time of its inception.

The progress of non-medical prescribing over the past few years has been phenomenal. From the prescribing of dressings through to the development of PGDs as a new mechanism to supply and administer medicines and the arrival of nurse and pharmacist independent prescribers, the face of non-medical prescribing has changed irrevocably and arguably for the benefit of patients with faster, safer and better access to medicines.

There remains one last block to faster access to medication. The Misuse of Drugs Act (currently under review), if amended, could allow independent prescribers throughout the UK to prescribe all controlled drugs, in all circumstances, within the prescriber's area of competence. Accordingly, it would release the whole *British National Formulary* to those competent and willing to prescribe from it. This would require some forward thinking within the Government, particularly from the Home Office who regulate the Misuse of Drugs Act. This final shift would enable even quicker, safer access to medicines in the near future by highly trained, competent independent prescribers.

Cases

Bolam v Friern Hospital Management Committee [1957] WLR 582

Bolitho v City and Hackney Health Authority [1997] 4 ALL ER 771 HL

Chester v Afshar [2004] UK HL 41 [2004] 3 WLR 927

Donoghue v Stevenson [1932] AC 562

Gascoigne v Ian Sheridan and Co and Latham [1994] 5 Med LR 437

McLennan v Newcastle Health Authority [1992] Med LR 215

Prendergast v Sam Dee [1989] Med LR 36

Re C (adult – refusal of medical treatment) [1994] 1 All ER 819

Re MB (adult – refusal of treatment) [1997] 2 FLR 426 CA

Scholendorff v Society of New York Hospital [1914] 105 NE 92

Statutes

Medicines Act 1968

Consumer Protection Act 1987

Medicinal Products: Prescription by Nurses etc. Act 1992

National Health Service Act 1997

Pharmaceutical Services Regulations 1994

Health and Social Care Act 2001

Mental Capacity Act 2005

Health Service Circular 2000/026

Home Office Circular 049/2003

Healthcare and Associated Professions Orders 2004/1756, 2004/1771

Medicines and Human Use (Prescribing) (Miscellaneous Amendments) Order 2006

References

Department of Health (1989). *Report of the Advisory Group on Nurse Prescribing (Crown Report).* London: HMSO.

Department of Health (1999). *Review of Prescribing, Supply and Administration of Medicines (Crown Report).* London: HMSO.

Department of Health (2003a). Patient Group Directions (PGDs). www.dh.gov.uk/nonmedical prescribing (accessed 1 June 2009).

Department of Health (2003b). Clinical Management Plans (CMPs) www.dh.gov.uk/ supplementaryprescribing (accessed 1 June 2009).

Department of Health (2006). *Medicine Matters. A Guide to the Prescribing, Supply and Administration of Medicines.* London: HMSO.

Department of Health and Social Security (1986). *Neighbourhood Nursing: a Focus for Care (Cumberlege Report).* London: HMSO.

Dimond, B. (2002). *Legal Aspects of Nursing* (third edition). Hemel Hempstead: Prentice Hall Publishing.

Gibson, B. (2001). Legal and professional accountability for nurse prescribing. In: Courtenay, M. (2001). *Current Issues in Nurse Prescribing*. London: GMM Ltd.

Griffith, R. (2006). Accountability and the nurse prescriber. *Nurse Prescriber* 4(9): 365–370.

Hendrick, J. (2000). *Law and Ethics in Nursing and Health Care*. Cheltenham: Stanley Thornes Publishers Ltd.

National Health Service Litigation Authority (2009). www.nhsla.com (accessed 1 June 2009).

National Patient Safety Agency (2007). *Safety in Doses: Medication Safety Incidents in the NHS*. London: NPSA.

National Prescribing Centre (2003). *Supplementary Prescribing. A Resource to Help Healthcare Professionals to Understand the Framework and Opportunities*. Liverpool: NPC.

Nursing and Midwifery Council (2005). *Circular 30/2005*. V100 nurse prescribers. London: NMC Publications.

Nursing and Midwifery Council (2006). *Standards of Proficiency for Nurse and Midwife Prescribers*. London: NMC Publications.

Nursing and Midwifery Council (2008). *The Code Standards of Conduct, Performance and Ethics for Nurses and Midwives*. London: NMC Publications.

Pennels, C. (1999). Nurse prescribing. When is prescribing not prescribing? *Nursing Times* 95(23 Suppl): 10–11.

Chapter 5

Ethical issues in independent and supplementary prescribing

John Adams

Ethics is concerned with the promotion of the high standards of conduct by which the public rightly expects healthcare practitioners to abide. The relationship between law and ethics in a democratic society should always be a close one. Legislators and judges create laws and legal decisions which can be enforced through the courts. Ethicists, on the other hand, spend their time reflecting on the implications of legal decisions and exploring the ways in which conduct can be guided by rational and coherent principles. There is a constant dialogue between legal scholars and ethicists as each seek to use the other's discipline to shed light on their own concerns. So it is not surprising that most textbooks for the healthcare professions, like this one, combine discussion of both law and ethics.

At the heart of ethics lies the process of reflecting on the dilemmas raised by professional practice. The contribution that ethics makes is to provide a range of possible theoretical tools or frameworks which may help to elucidate the issues that are at stake, and which may provide consistent guidance on which principles should be given the most weight. Ethics does not, therefore, provide a simple system which will provide the 'right' answer when faced with any dilemma in prescribing practice. It is the starting point for the debate rather than its neat and tidy conclusion. Professional practice in healthcare in the modern world requires the balancing of complex competing needs and interests. Practitioners' responses to this kind of ethical exploration and debate depend to a large extent on how useful they feel this process of reflection to be.

The authority to prescribe raises a range of important ethical concerns, such as the need to obtain informed consent, the requirement to respect confidentiality and decisions over the allocation of scarce resources. At the heart of ethical considerations of prescribing is the imbalance of power between the prescriber and the patient. Where one person has power over another, the potential for abuse of that situation always exists, and the power to control access to potentially important medication requires frequent review and reflection.

Ethical frameworks

Subjective ethics

Many people would argue that ethical decision making is essentially a simple matter of listening to our conscience. They believe that when confronted with an ethical dilemma, we all know instinctively what the 'right' course of action is. No-one would want to deny the power of conscience. Over the course of many centuries, brave individuals have felt compelled to follow the dictates of their conscience, even at great cost to themselves. Even today, much 'whistle-blowing' activity in the health service is motivated by the subjective guidance of an individual conscience. So while not wishing to diminish the undoubted power of individual subjective approaches to decision making in ethics, it must also be recognised that they have some serious shortcomings. The fundamental problem posed by subjective approaches to ethics is the potential for a lack of consistency, with an absence of agreed principles on which to rely for guidance. If a prescriber announces that they feel free to ignore the requirement for patient confidentiality or that their conscience tells them to dispense with informed consent, discussion generally proves fruitless. As the saying goes, 'there is no reasoning with conscience'. So while the ability to follow the guidance of conscience is a highly desirable characteristic in any healthcare professional, it is not sufficient on its own. Objective external standards are necessary in order to ensure that practitioners have an outside frame of reference against which to judge their actions.

Paternalism

Paternalism (literally 'acting like a father', by implementing decisions which are felt to be in the patient's best interest, but without obtaining prior informed consent) has been the dominant tradition in Western medicine. Until comparatively recently, healthcare professionals believed that it was their role to decide on courses of treatment without necessarily gaining the consent of the patient. While it is easy to blame the various professions concerned, and to regard paternalism as evidence of an oppressive medical conspiracy, it is probably more correct to see it as expressing the preference of most patients at that time to be told, rather than to be asked. The last 50 years, however, have seen a decisive shift in public opinion against medical paternalism and in favour of informed consent. This fundamental shift in our culture has several roots. Most people now regard decisions about what happens to their own body as among the most important they are ever called upon to take. So they are naturally unwilling to delegate them to health service professionals. Secondly, the dominance of consumerism in all other walks of life has an inevitable impact upon healthcare. As we expect to select from the supermarket precisely what we want, when we require it, it is not surprising that increasingly 'consumerist' attitudes are permeating the health service. Recent scandals involving poor standards of performance by healthcare professionals are only likely to accelerate this trend. Finally, as prescribers are concerned about compliance or concordance with medication regimes, accurate adherence to them is presumably more likely to be achieved if the patient has been fully involved in the decision-making process.

Having outlined some of the shortcomings of traditional medical paternalism, it is important to stress that the opposite extreme, laissez-faire practice, is equally inappropriate. The prescriber who said to all their patients, 'Just tell me what you want and I will prescribe it for you', would not be acting ethically. The prescriber has a responsibility to assess each patient's needs and to recommend a course of treatment, if that is felt to be appropriate. This recommendation will include a willingness to discuss possible side effects, and the pros and cons of other potential treatment options. In situations where the patient is unable to take part in the decision-making process, because of a reduced conscious level or a confusional state, for example, society would expect a prescriber to make decisions in what are genuinely felt to be the patient's best interests.One of the key principles underlying the Mental Capacity Act 2005 is that any act done to a person who lacks capacity must be in their best interests. The website of the Office of the Public Guardian provides guidance on the issues to be considered (http://www.publicguardian.gov.uk/index.htm).

Deontological ethics

There is a long tradition of adopting concepts from philosophy in order to illuminate ethical discussion. Deontology (from the Greek word for duty or obligation) is the name given to a school of thought in philosophy which emphasises that there are certain fixed duties which everyone ought to undertake. Most of the great religions of the world promote a deontological approach to ethics. One example, shared by Judaism and Christianity, is the Ten Commandments. The statement 'thou shalt not kill' lays down an ethical standard which does not grant exceptions, or suggest that the consequences of an action in any particular situation should be taken into account. The strength of this kind of approach to ethics is that it encourages all practitioners to aspire to an equally high standard of conduct. Patients can feel confidence that ethical principles will be adhered to whatever the circumstances in which they find themselves. The main weakness, on the other hand, of the deontological approach to ethics is that it is inflexible and may not take particular circumstances into account. To give an extreme example, if a gunman takes a ward full of patients and staff hostage and threatens to kill them all, police marksmen may feel justified in breaking the prohibition against murder in order to save the maximum number of lives. As no healthcare system in the world provides all the resources which every patient may require, healthcare professionals are always faced with the necessity of deciding priorities rather than following unchanging duties. Cash-limited drug budgets present a good example of the kind of prioritisation decisions that have to take place. The prescriber is simply unable to meet every need that could be met.

Immanuel Kant (1724–1804), a professor of philosophy at Königsberg University in Prussia, developed an influential approach to deontological ethics based upon human reason and religious belief. The central tenet in his approach to ethics is that human beings should always be regarded as ends in themselves, rather than as means to an end. One could imagine a situation in which a pharmaceutical researcher is so convinced that a new drug will benefit humanity that he becomes careless about the suffering of the people taking part in the trials of early versions of the medication. Kant's ethical principle reminds us that all human beings have equal value.

> Immanuel Kant emphasised that to be ethical, principles should be applicable in all similar situations: he wrote that we should 'act upon a maxim that can also hold as a universal law' (Wood 1999).

When resources are limited, there is always the temptation to make exceptions for special cases: for colleagues; for patients who seem particularly needy or who tug at the heart strings – the list could go on and on. Kant reminds us that fairness and equal rights should lie at the heart of ethically defensible decision making. A practitioner with the power to prescribe needs to reflect long and hard about providing something for one person or group which would not normally be available for all.

Utilitarian ethics

In the nineteenth century, leading thinkers turned away from deontological ethics on the grounds that its inflexible rules did not provide guidance for the dilemmas which people face in everyday life. In the place of duty-based ethics, two British philosophers, Jeremy Bentham (1748–1832) and John Stuart Mill (1806–1873), developed a highly influential approach to practical ethics which was based upon the idea of evaluating the consequences of an ethical decision. In their view, the decision which maximised happiness was the ethically correct one to take. The everyday usefulness of this approach was emphasised by their calling it 'utilitarian ethics'. In place of happiness, modern utilitarians tend to advocate decisions which result in 'the greatest good for the greatest number'.

Utilitarian ethics can be found being used to justify actions in all areas of the modern health service. Triage procedures in the accident and emergency department are designed to ensure that patients in most need are treated first. Hospital wards are also generally run on utilitarian principles. Patients deemed to have the greatest clinical need are generally nursed in beds nearest the nurses' station, and receive the most attention. Most countries in the developed world use waiting lists for treatment which give priority to those whose clinical need is judged to be greatest.

In situations where there is agreement about where the 'greatest good' lies, utilitarian ethics command wide acceptance. So most people would agree that the saving of life in the emergency situation takes precedence over other issues. Most people stop their car to allow the ambulance with the blue flashing light to overtake. Similarly, there is a general acceptance that patients with severe trauma should receive priority treatment in the accident and emergency department.

> Utilitarianism provides the classic justification for devoting scarce resources to where they will do the greatest good. Drug budgets are finite, while demand is increasing all the time. It is therefore no surprise that rationing continues to dominate debates about the future direction of health policy (Klein 2007).

The fact that utilitarian justifications are given for decisions taken throughout the health service means that this approach to ethics can soon come to be regarded as 'the obvious way of doing things', and so beyond debate. This makes it particularly important that utilitarianism is not adopted uncritically and that due weight is given to its potential weaknesses as an ethical philosophy. The main criticism concerns those who lose out when utilitarian criteria are applied. There are losers as well as winners when such judgements are made. Historically, some groups always had a low priority in the competition for scarce National Health Service (NHS) resources – for example, older people, people with a learning disability and those who were mentally ill. So the question must be posed: what about the needs of the low-priority, low-status patient? The recent development of an NHS culture of inspections, targets, audit and National Service Frameworks can be seen as an attempt to ensure that utilitarian excesses are moderated and that resources are devoted to all. A second weakness of utilitarian ethics is that it depends upon an ability to predict the future. Indeed, utilitarianism is sometimes referred to as a 'consequentialist' approach to ethics, as the utilitarian must weigh up the likely consequences of possible actions, and choose the option which maximises the happiness or the good. Yet predicting the outcome of a particular clinical decision can be difficult. The continuing development of evidence-based practice should enable practitioners to make more informed judgements about likely outcomes.

Summary

From the perspective of philosophical ethics, the prescriber can be portrayed as trapped between two opposing forces: deontological and utilitarian ethics.

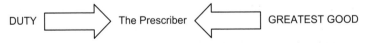

On the one hand, the healthcare professional feels duty-bound to meet all the needs that patients present. On the other hand are the pressures exerted by budgetary limits and a health service which often demands that needs are prioritised.

A principles-based approach

While deontological and utilitarian approaches to ethics may provide the context in which decisions are taken, practitioners generally feel the need for ethical guidance which is more specifically related to the clinical dilemmas that they face in everyday practice. The most influential figures in the biomedical field are the two American ethicists, Tom L. Beauchamp and James F. Childress. They argue that it is possible to identify four key ethical principles in the medical tradition – respect for autonomy, non-maleficence (that is, avoiding causing harm), beneficence (seeking to do good to patients) and justice, which they supplement with four 'rules', veracity, privacy, confidentiality and fidelity (Beauchamp and Childress 2009).

(1) Respect for autonomy

It is no coincidence that Beauchamp and Childress place 'respect for autonomy' first in their consideration of the principles which should guide ethical decision making. As we have seen, most patients today reject paternalistic attitudes on the part of healthcare professionals. Both the legal and ethical dimensions of informed consent rest on a similar set of procedures. There is an underlying assumption that the patient will have the intellectual capacity to understand the issues that are to be decided, the ability to decide between the various options presented and a memory of what was decided. The role of the prescriber is to outline the choices to be made, provide sufficient background information including that on any side effects of the proposed treatment and likely effects of non-treatment, and to recommend a course of action. Even though this approach has become the expected norm, it is easy to find patients who can describe prescribing encounters which have fallen a long way short of this standard.

Recent emphasis on the central importance of obtaining informed consent can sometimes lead practitioners to assume that patients *must* take part in the decisions concerning their treatment. But if we are serious about respecting autonomy, then presumably we must respect a patient's right not to choose that course of treatment. It is clear that there are some patients who genuinely do not want to take part in such decision making and would rather the prescriber acted in their best interests, but without their involvement. This is sometimes felt to be a characteristic of some older patients who are believed to be more comfortable with a situation in which 'the prescriber knows best'. However, it is apparent that there are patients of all ages who take such a stance, and respect for their autonomy means that the prescriber should support their choice.

> Consider a scenario in which a patient presents at the clinic with a sore throat and requests a course of antibiotic treatment in order to cure it. After a careful history has been taken, and an examination carried out, the prescriber concludes that a prescription for a course of antibiotic therapy would be inappropriate. The patient says, 'You are just trying to save money from the drug budget.' The prescriber calmly explains the evidence base for the decision. The patient continues to demand a prescription for an antibiotic.

Such is the power of consumerism in our society, with its slogan 'the customer is always right', that some patients have problems in modifying this approach when faced with healthcare settings. As important as 'respect for autonomy' is in current ethical thought, few ethicists would argue that patient choice should override all other considerations. However, while such situations may prove difficult for the current prescriber, the development of information technology looks set to pose even greater challenges in the future. The increasing availability of medical information on the internet and the web-based international trade in pharmaceutical products are likely to create major issues for both the individual prescriber and the national regulatory authorities in the not too distant future.

In most healthcare settings, and on most occasions, patients follow the advice given to them by the staff. This can soon lead to the complacent belief that 'respect for autonomy' raises few issues. Yet it may only be when a patient makes what the staff consider to be a 'foolish' decision that the concept of autonomy and its limits is fully explored. Our society is gradually becoming more accepting of such patient decisions. Refusing to accept medication may shorten life, but society now generally accepts such a decision in a competent adult.

(2) Non-maleficence

The principle of non-maleficence means that the prescriber has an active duty to avoid causing harm to patients. This concept is sometimes encountered in the form of the Latin phrase, 'primum non nocere' – above all, do no harm – and some clinicians regard it as the central concept in medical ethics. Medication can have seriously harmful consequences, and for some patients may even prove to be fatal. So the prescriber clearly has an ethical duty to consider carefully any harmful effects that the prescribed medication may have. Therefore it could be argued that maintaining professional competence through evidence-based practice is an ethical imperative as well as a professional one. However, non-maleficence can never be an absolute requirement as all drugs have potentially harmful side effects, and a desire to avoid all harm would inevitably mean that no prescriptions were ever written. So the challenge for the prescriber seeking to prescribe ethically is to judge which risks, and which levels of risk, are appropriate in any given clinical situation.

> The current emphasis on the unwanted side effects of medication can sometimes have an unfortunate influence upon decision making by patients. I used to visit a sprightly woman of 90, who had a store of vivid memories about the history of local towns and villages. As she had severe hypertension, her GP had prescribed anti-hypertensive medication for her. Whenever I visited, she used to show me the leaflet enclosed in the box. She would unroll it like an ancient scroll and solemnly intone the list of frightening conditions of which she was warned. It did indeed appear that these innocuous-looking tablets threatened just about every ill known to humankind. Being struck by lightning seemed to be just about the only risk not to be increased. So my advice to her to follow the prescriber's instructions fell on deaf ears. When feeling particularly unwell, she took a few of the tablets, but as soon as she started to feel better they were discontinued – 'because they can harm you, dear – just look at what it says in this leaflet!'

(3) Beneficence

Beneficence – the duty to do good – has always been central to the role of the healthcare professional. It is a dynamic process which actively seeks out the most appropriate treatment for the patient. Therefore beneficence is underpinned by regular professional updating so that the most effective therapies can be prescribed. While few would argue with the importance of beneficence when expressed in this way, the risk is that it shades over into paternalism: 'I know what is good for you: trust me, I'm a prescriber'.

(4) Justice

Philosophers since at least the time of Aristotle have argued that human beings have an innate regard for justice. Fairness, however, requires restraint on the part of some who could grab more than their fair share. When drug budgets are limited, the issue of justice towards patients is an important and controversial one. As priorities have to be set, one approach is that local trusts are best placed to distribute their resources in an equitable manner. As this will inevitably mean that a drug or treatment will be available in one area but not another, the campaigning cry immediately goes up that this is 'postcode prescribing'. Both National Service Frameworks and the National Institute for Health and Clinical Excellence (NICE) are part of the policy imperative to ensure uniformity across the NHS. How local priorities and national requirements can be reconciled has yet to be elucidated.

(a) Veracity

Veracity, or truthfulness, is an essential component of informed consent and hence of respect for autonomy. Asking a patient whether they would choose the red tablets or the purple ones, without further information, does not show respect for autonomy. While everyone supports the principle of veracity, putting it into practice provides major scope for ethical dilemmas. Issues around how much should be told, to whom, and in what circumstances, creates continuing difficulty for healthcare professionals. As we saw earlier, complete information on side effects may cause the patient to stop taking the medication. But who is to say what is 'enough'? Even starker dilemmas are raised if bad news is to be conveyed.

(b) Privacy

Elevating the concept of privacy to a key role in ethical debate represents a new and challenging departure from the traditions of medical ethics. The key issue here is what information a patient should share with a healthcare professional, and what can be kept secret. The concept of patient privacy forms a thought-provoking challenge to some current concepts of 'holistic assessment and care planning'. Ranging across the '12 activities of living' (Roper et al. 2000), to collect information about a patient's lifestyle far removed from the presenting problem, may have major implications for the desire for privacy. Even though the NHS has in the past set little store by patient privacy in its communal wards and clinics, some areas of privacy have existed for many years. One example is treatment in a clinic for sexually transmitted diseases. The records of such treatment episodes are kept separate from general hospital records, and so patients' privacy is maintained if treatment is sought for other types of condition. Such a system operates effectively when paper records are involved, but increasing automation poses real threats to privacy. The development of an electronic patient record needs to take such concerns into account if it is to command public trust (Pagliari et al. 2007).

(c) Confidentiality

Modern medical treatment almost always requires communication of patient details between departments, teams and individuals, if the optimum level of care is to be provided. This immediately undermines the old ideal of patient secrets being retained by one doctor. So health service organisations must continually review their measures in place to protect patient confidentiality.

(d) Fidelity

Fidelity is concerned with faithfully maintaining the duty to care, even in difficult circumstances. The NHS and its staff have a generally laudable tradition of maintaining treatment for patients or clients who have been stigmatised or even rejected by the rest of society. A local television news programme recently reported on the plight of a group of traveller families in great need, from whom all contact with official bodies had been withdrawn. The only 'professional' who continued to offer support was a health visitor. Her ongoing care for the children and their parents demonstrated fidelity in action. Prescribers are likely to have frequent contact with patients who exhibit challenging behaviour or who are stigmatised for some reason. Possession of the power of control over medication inevitably places the prescriber on society's 'front line'. The concept of fidelity provides a reminder of society's expectation of the manner in which the power is to be exercised.

Codes of conduct

One of the earliest statements of ethical principles in medicine was the Hippocratic Oath. Like all ethical codes, it combines timeless precepts with ideas relevant only to the time and society which created it. It advocates doing good and avoiding harm, and not taking advantage of the vulnerable, but it also forbids doctors from undertaking surgical procedures. This reflects a historical context in which educated physicians looked down upon the artisans who combined the practice of surgery with bloodletting and maintaining a barber's shop. Many of the Hippocratic precepts, such as 'doing good' and 'avoiding harm', can still be found in modern codes of conduct for healthcare professionals. The principles-based approach of Beauchamp and Childress (2009) has also been highly influential in the development of such codes. One example is *The Code: Standards of Conduct, Performance and Ethics for Nurses and Midwives* (NMC 2008). Many of its clauses can be mapped against their principles and rules. For example:

Respect for autonomy:

- You must ensure that you gain consent before you begin any treatment or care.
- You must respect and support people's rights to accept or decline treatment and care.

Non-maleficence

- You must act without delay if you believe that you, a colleague or anyone else may be putting someone at risk.

Beneficence

- Work with others to protect and promote the health and wellbeing of those in your care, their families and carers, and the wider community.

Justice

- You must demonstrate a personal and professional commitment to equality and diversity.

Veracity

- Be open and honest, act with integrity and uphold the reputation of your profession.

Confidentiality

- You must respect people's right to confidentiality.
- You must ensure people are informed about how and why information is shared by those who will be providing their care.

Fidelity

- You must not allow someone's complaint to prejudice the care you provide for them.

A similar exercise can be carried out with the *Code of Ethics for Pharmacists and Pharmacy Technicians*, published by the Royal Pharmaceutical Society of Great Britain (RPSGB 2007), which can be downloaded from their website (http://www.rpsgb.org.uk). The code lays down seven principles, which require pharmacists and pharmacy technicians to:

1. Make the care of patients your first concern.
2. Exercise your professional judgement in the interests of patients and the public.

3. Show respect for others.
4. Encourage patients to participate in decisions about their care.
5. Develop your professional knowledge and competence.
6. Be honest and trustworthy.
7. Take responsibility for your working practices.

The prescriber and the pharmaceutical companies

The attainment of prescribing rights will inevitably bring the individual prescriber into close contact with pharmaceutical companies and their representatives. The ethical aspects of existing links between the industry and medical practitioners are widely debated. Some argue that doctors need to 'disentangle' themselves from this relationship, while others advocate a continuing dialogue between the two parties (Moynihan 2003a; 2003b; Wager 2003). In the United Kingdom, the activities of pharmaceutical companies are subject to the Association of the British Pharmaceutical Industry (ABPI) *Code of Practice for the Pharmaceutical Industry* (2008), and all prescribers need to familiarise themselves with its provisions. Complaints about the conduct of pharmaceutical companies can be made to the Prescription Medicines Code of Practice Authority (PMCPA), and the latest edition of their *Code of Practice Review* can be accessed via their website (http://www.pmcpa.org.uk).

What is your opinion of this advertisement?

Are you a prescriber?
In need of some winter sunshine?
If you can answer 'YES' to these two questions,
let Whamo Pharmaceuticals whisk you
and your partner to a 5-star hotel in
Monaco
for a short product briefing
(…then shop 'til you drop!)

Clause 19.1 of the *Code of Practice for the Pharmaceutical Industry* (ABPI 2008), governing meetings and hospitality, is relevant here. It states that:

- 'Meetings must be held in appropriate venues conducive to the main purpose of the event.'
- 'Hospitality must be strictly limited to the main purpose of the event and must be secondary to the purpose of the meeting, i.e. subsistence only.'
- 'The costs involved must not exceed that level which the recipients would normally adopt when paying for themselves.'
- '(Hospitality) must not extend beyond members of the health professions or appropriate administrative staff.'

As, on the face of it, this advertisement appears to offer hospitality which contravenes all four elements of the clause, referral to the PMCPA would seem to be appropriate.

While attention inevitably tends to focus on those isolated instances when the code is disregarded, the reality is that pharmaceutical companies make a major contribution to educational activities of all kinds. Attendance at local educational meetings, which may receive sponsorship from pharmaceutical companies, can provide an important source of information about developments in prescribing. The following advertisement appears to indicate a worthwhile meeting with an appropriate level of hospitality.

'Current trends in asthma care'
Lunchtime lecture
by
Professor M. Fulbourn FRCP
Location: The Interchange Motel, Loamstone
Sandwich lunch provided
Sponsors: Whamo Pharmaceuticals

When the ethics of a prescriber receiving gifts or hospitality from a pharmaceutical company are discussed, attention tends to focus upon any potential influence that this may have upon the behaviour and attitudes of the prescriber. Yet surely this is to ignore the most important participant in the encounter: the patient. Little research has been done on the attitudes of patients towards prescribers receiving gifts from the pharmaceutical industry. In one American study, a survey was conducted to compare the attitudes of prescribing physicians with those of patients attending their hospitals, on whether it was appropriate to accept gifts and whether this would be likely to influence prescribing behaviour (Gibbons et al. 1998). The results indicated that patients found gifts less appropriate and more influential than did their physicians. As the legal profession discovered many years ago, 'justice must not only be done, it must be seen to be done'. Transparency is a key requirement in decision-making processes if the public is to retain confidence in those decisions. In exactly the same way, a prescriber needs to be constantly reviewing how his or her acceptance of gifts may be perceived by patients.

Picture the scene. You are a patient arriving at a clinic for a consultation. Once inside the consulting room, the first thing you notice is that the handsome desk set and blotter carry a slogan from Whamo Pharmaceuticals. As your eyes rove around the room, you cannot help noticing that the same logo is also displayed on the year planner on the wall and on the prescriber's smart document case lying on the floor. Having assessed your condition thoroughly, the healthcare professional explains that you need a prescription for the new drug, Whamo-lite. As the pen (guess who provided it!) moves effortlessly across the prescription pad, how much confidence do you feel in the independence of the prescriber's judgement?

Research ethics and the prescriber

Pharmaceutical research is a major generator of the research activity in the NHS, and much of it involves the crucial participation of prescribers. So all prescribers need to be aware of the main features of the NHS system in place to review research protocols in order to provide ethical safeguards for patients and staff. The cornerstone of the system is the Local Research Ethics Committee (LREC) which regulates research within a defined geographical area. LRECs were first established in the 1960s and their procedures were set out in health service guidance published in 1991 (HSG (91) 5). Originally, the area covered by an LREC was relatively small and so major studies conducted by pharmaceutical companies required detailed negotiations with numerous LRECs. In 1997, a new tier of regulation for large studies, the Multi-Centre Research Ethics Committee, was set up (HSG (97) 23). Policy in the area of research ethics is guided by the document, *Research Governance Framework for Health and Social Care: Second Edition* (DoH 2005). The co-ordination of this policy in England is being undertaken by the

National Research Ethics Service, which maintains an informative website (http://www.nres.npsa.nhs.uk). Similar arrangements concerning the ethical regulation of research are in place for Wales, Scotland and Northern Ireland. It is a requirement that research involving patients, service users, care professionals or volunteers, or their organs, tissue or data, is reviewed independently to ensure it meets ethical standards (DoH 2005).

Conclusion

Recent well-publicised scandals in the medical and nursing professions have damaged public confidence in the ethical standards displayed by healthcare professionals, and in the ability of the professions to maintain ethical standards (DoH/Ho 2007). Some of these scandals, such as that concerning the GP Dr Harold Shipman, have involved the misuse of prescribed medication for criminal purposes. Almost inevitably, the cry is taken up by the mass media to demand that 'healthcare professionals must have more teaching on ethics'. Sadly, no amount of reflection on ethics is likely to have stopped those who have such murderous inclinations. In addition, when such stories break, calls are inevitably made for the closer supervision of prescribers. While there is no doubt some merit in reviewing the regulations, there are finite limits to what such supervision can achieve. In the final analysis, society has no alternative but to trust prescribers (O'Neill 2002). So the responsibility for fostering that trust lies with all who have the authority to prescribe.

References

Association of British Pharmaceutical Industries (2008). *ABPI Code of Practice for the Pharmaceutical Industry.* http://www.abpi.org.uk/publications/pdfs/pmpca_code2008.pdf (accessed 10 December 2009).

Beauchamp, T.L., Childress, J.F. (2009). *Principles of Biomedical Ethics.* (sixth edition). New York: Oxford University Press.

Department of Health (2005). *Research Governance Framework for Health and Social Care* (second edition). London: Department of Health.

Department of Health/Home Office (2007). *Learning from Tragedy, Keeping Patients Safe. Cm 7014.* London: The Stationery Office.

Gibbons, R.V., Landry, F.J., Blouch, D.L. et al. (1998). A comparison of physicians' and patients' attitudes toward pharmaceutical industry gifts. *J Gen Int Med 13*: 151–154.

Klein, R. (2007). Rationing in the NHS. *BMJ 334*: 1068–1069.

Moynihan, R. (2003a). *Who pays for the pizza? Redefining the relationships between doctors and drug companies. 1*: Entanglement. *BMJ 326*: 1189–1192.

Moynihan, R. (2003b). *Who pays for the pizza? Redefining the relationships between doctors and drug companies. 2: Disentanglement. BMJ 326*: 1193–1196.

Nursing and Midwifery Council (2008). *The Code: Standards of Conduct, Performance and Ethics for Nurses and Midwives.* London: NMC.

O'Neill, O. (2002). *Autonomy and Trust in Bioethics.* Cambridge: Cambridge University Press.

Pagliari, C., Detmer, D., Singleton, P. (2007). Potential of electronic personal health records. *BMJ 335*: 330–333.

Roper, N., Logan, W.W., Tierney, A.J. (2000). *The Roper-Logan-Tierney Model of Nursing: Based on Activities of Living.* Edinburgh: Churchill Livingstone.

Royal Pharmaceutical Society of Great Britain (2007). *Code of Ethics for Pharmacists and Pharmacy Technicians.* London: RPSGB.

Wager, E. (2003). How to dance with porcupines: rules and guidelines on doctors' relations with drug companies. *BMJ 326*: 1196–1198.

Wood, A.W. (1999). *Kant's Ethical Thought.* Cambridge: Cambridge University Press.

6 Psychology and sociology of prescribing

Tom Walley and Robin Williams

Why do doctors and other health professionals prescribe medicines? Why do patients want to take medicines? The simple answers to these questions can all be framed in terms of a biomedical model of the patient presenting with an illness and the prescriber trying to provide the means to help the patient get better. But this is only a partial truth, and really, prescribing is a more complex social interaction. Prescribing can be a means to a variety of ends. Unless we understand this, and understand why prescribers and patients behave as they do, we cannot understand prescribing. What is termed 'irrational prescribing' can often be explained, and by this understanding, we can work towards helping both prescribers and patients make the best use of medicines.

This chapter concerns itself with the multiplicity of non-biomedical reasons why patients may or may not receive a prescription. These lie partly in the psychology of the interaction between the individual prescriber and patient, but partly in the societies or cultures, professional, ethnic, local or even national, within which each operates; these two are so interwoven that they are best considered side by side.

In this chapter, we will talk a lot about doctor behaviour. This is because almost all of the research so far is about how doctors, rather than other professions, behave in relation to prescribing. But the reasons why doctors prescribe are the same as those which will drive the prescribing of other professions, and to assume that nurses or pharmacists will prescribe better or be less influenced by these pressures because they spend longer with the patient and so won't fall into all of the problems discussed here, is simply wrong.

Sociological models

It might help if we briefly gave a description of various medical sociological theories or models that have been developed to explain prescribing behaviour.

Lay belief system: Nurses, doctors, pharmacists and many healthcare professionals have beliefs firmly lodged in what can be termed 'Western modern medicine' – a belief in medicine as a science rather than a superstition, in the principles of evidence-based medicine, in physical rather than magical causes for illness, and conversely in pharmacological cures rather than placebo. But people, namely most patients, work outside this close-knit professional group and have widely differing ideas. These ideas do not fit neatly into the scientific belief system. The range of these ideas is quite staggering and varies significantly among social groups within different cultures. These beliefs strongly determine when patients seek medical care, their expectations about receiving medicines and the type of treatments which they seek.

The sick role: This was first described by Talcott Parsons back in 1951. The sick role is deemed a temporary state wherein the patient cedes control of his life to others, usually to medics and nurses, on the grounds of ill health. This may be some form of global ill health requiring, for instance, hospital admission or a much narrower role, such as high blood pressure.

The person then becomes a patient, who is expected to accept and follow the advice of these professionals. At the same time, an individual who enters the sick role then becomes privileged and protected, and is then able to shed some of their responsibilities, such as the need to go to work or turn up for school.

Sanctioning and legitimising: The doctor has traditionally acted as gatekeeper into this sick role, but increasingly professionals other than doctors are also involved. For many patients, a prescription is the ticket for entry into or to confirm this role. It is the external legitimisation of some illnesses, and conversely if a doctor refuses a prescription, friends or relatives may assume 'there's nothing much wrong with him', i.e. the legitimisation has been denied. For many patients, it is as if the doctor has refused to acknowledge their illness. The patient may therefore be very resentful of such a refusal and the prescriber may not be well accepted by the patient when trying to explain, for instance, that antibiotics do not work for viral illnesses.

Doctors act as gatekeepers not only to medical care, but also to many aspects of social care. Doctors enable people to take time off work or school. They may enable access to sick pay or other benefits. Society tends to define the boundaries, and a patient who the doctor deems unfit for these privileges might be considered a malingerer. This is a very powerful position for the professions. Prescribing might be one expression of sanctioning this process.

Medicalisation: More and more areas seem to become subject to the control and the jurisdiction of medicine. Doctors and others may encourage this to extend their professional power. The medical supervision of the natural acts of childbirth or the menopause might be seen as examples of this. People such as Illich, author of the famous book *Medical Nemesis* (Illich 1981), believe this whole process has gone too far.

Prescribing responsibility is an expression of this power. Drugs may become part of this medicalisation, as the pharmaceutical industry seeks new markets to extend its profits. For instance, is a disease increasingly defined by the fact that there is a drug available to treat the problem? This is perhaps most apparent when we think about so called 'lifestyle drugs' such as sildenafil (Viagra) or orlistat (Xenical) (Gilbert et al. 2000). While recognising that obesity is a serious problem which causes a lot of morbidity, when does it move from a matter of personal choice (to eat too much, to exercise too little) to a medical matter in which the patient cedes control to the professionals? To what extent did this develop when there were drugs available to treat the condition? There is no easy answer to this question, which is often rooted in cultural perceptions of what illness is. For instance, the French consume vast amounts of medication (about 55 prescriptions per head per year), while the Dutch take very little by comparison (around 5–6 prescriptions per year; in the UK, the average is 11–12 per year). This is not explained by the French being vastly more unhealthy than the Dutch, but clearly the French have different ideas about what is appropriate medical care.

Opposing this growing medicalisation is a counterculture of patients becoming more assertive in taking more control of their own health and being involved in their own treatments. The chapter on concordance will say much more about this. There is clearly a balance to be struck here between self-care and care from health professionals, and the balance varies from culture to culture, and from patient to patient.

Why *do* doctors (and others) prescribe?

As we said in the introduction, this question could be answered simply in a biomedical way about illness, the pathophysiology of the illness and a desire to use the pharmacological effect of a drug to improve the patient's condition. Harris and co-workers (Harris et al. 1990) described this as the 'respectable' answer, but found a lot of evidence that doctors often prescribe even when they anticipate no real medical benefit from the drug. They identify a range of non-biomedical reasons why doctors prescribe:

- To avoid doing something else (like referring a patient to hospital or another service).
- To maintain contact. This may seem to be an odd point but remember that a GP has to work with a patient to improve the patient's health over many years. If he antagonises a patient over a refused prescription for an antibiotic, the relationship may fail and undermine what the doctor might want to do about long-term management of the patient's diabetes or ischaemic heart disease. In this situation, many doctors would let the occasional (biomedically 'inappropriate') prescription pass. This is not an excuse for prescribing anything to everyone, as again there has to be a balance. The occasional prescription in this way may leave the door open for the patient to return with the same or other problems, while a cold refusal of a prescription may seem to slam the door in the patient's face.
- To temporise and gain time. Often the diagnosis is not clear in early disease. So prescribing may allow time for the disease process to become clear or, if it is a self-limiting illness, to go away. This temporising is part of the first two points – to avoid referring the patient perhaps needlessly, while keeping the process under observation. It may also be important to allow patients time to understand their own diseases or conditions.
- For some doctors, this is a way of dealing with uncertainty: in general practice in particular, the diagnosis is often unclear and the doctor responds to his or her 'best formulation' of what is wrong with the patient and acts accordingly. Some doctors find such uncertainty very difficult, and handle it by making firm (but sometimes unwarranted) diagnoses, and then prescribing.
- To satisfy an urge to give. The patient has come to the doctor with some distress. There may be a very human feeling that the doctor has to give something to the patient out of compassion, even if what is given is inappropriate. A doctor may see a single mother with two children living on the 12th floor of a high rise tower block where vandalism means the lifts are often out of action. The patient might complain of anxiety and depression, and who might not be anxious or depressed in such circumstances? Prescribing anything may be considered inappropriate – this is after all not a medical but a social problem. Nevertheless, the human urge to support the patient in some way and not reject the patient's distress may lead to a prescription for an anxiolytic or an antidepressant. There may even be some rationalising as to the reasons why the prescription was written, so that it apparently fits into the respectable biomedical model.

The ability to empathise with the patient may be a key factor here. In one study, Howie (1976) showed doctors pictures of sore throats with brief vignettes of the patient and clinical circumstances, and asked the doctors whether they would prescribe antibiotics or not. In fact the pictures and the vignettes were randomly paired and it was not the clinical features which determined the decision to prescribe but factors such as time of day, previous experience with this particular patient and often the social standing of the patient (more likely to prescribe an antibiotic for the child of a barrister than a labourer). We have conducted informal studies in the same way with nurses and pharmacists: those who were mothers were particularly given to prescribing for children, and the younger subjects were particularly keen to prescribe for a vignette that involved a young student coming up to examinations. So when the potential prescriber empathised with the patient's situation it elicited a prescription more easily.

Others have expanded this list of reasons for prescribing considerably and some of these suggestions are even further removed from the 'respectable':

- To terminate the consultation (how often do some doctors reach for the prescription pad as soon as the patient walks in the door?).
- To maintain the role of the doctor (is this being undermined by increasing availability of over-the-counter drugs and nurse or pharmacist prescribing?).
- To use the power of the placebo effect (see below).
- To legitimise the patient's illness, as we have talked about above.
- To earn money in pharmaceutical industry-sponsored post-marketing surveillance studies.
- To avoid medicolegal fears, as a feature of defensive medicine ('I might be sued if I don't prescribe an antibiotic here and something terrible, however rare or unlikely, happens').
- To avoid being called out (or to pay for the deputising service). This is said to be the reason for a lot of Friday afternoon antibiotic prescriptions when the doctor prescribes because he won't be available to monitor the condition over the weekend. There is an element of peer pressure here for the doctor – who may fear criticism from colleagues if they get called out to deal with a deteriorating patient over a weekend.
- Habit or previous experience – we are all heavily influenced by what happened the last time we did something or prescribed something. If a patient had a severe adverse effect, we are not going to prescribe *that* drug again no matter how rare the adverse reaction is.
- Precedent ('Dr X always prescribes drug Y for me when I have this…').

And so on. You could think of lots more reasons from your personal observations or practice.

Is prescribing for these non-medical reasons, or allowing your decision to prescribe be influenced by any of these, rational? From a strict biomedical standpoint perhaps not, but from many other points it might be. Again there is a balance to be struck here. For most of us, the balance we would like to achieve lies heavily but not exclusively on the biomedical side. But we cannot ignore the other reasons for prescribing and should reflect honestly on our own practice to consider where our point of balance is. Perhaps the worst position is to fool ourselves that we are always acting on the biomedical side when in fact we are responding to other pressures.

Sometimes we rationalise these influences and create more legitimate reasons for prescribing, and often it is not black and white any more than diagnoses are – these influences may play their biggest role when the biomedical decision to prescribe or not prescribe is marginal, rather than when to prescribe at all would be thought inappropriate. But the doctor who tells himself that he is prescribing antibiotics for what he knows are viral infections 'in case of a bacterial superinfection' is deluding himself – in effect prescribing a dual placebo, both for the patient and for himself.

Other influences on the doctor

We will look at the patient's influence on the doctor later but to be complete, we need to consider some other influences directly on the doctor outside the consultation (Bradley 1991).

- Colleagues: senior colleagues ('opinion leaders') are very influential in encouraging the issuing of a prescription or not in particular circumstances – medical teachers have particular responsibilities here. Peer pressure is a very important factor, as most of us do not like to be too out of line with what everyone else is doing. This factor is often used either by pharmaceutical companies or by health authorities to influence prescribing.

- Pharmaceutical companies are very influential, both for good and for bad. They can be a valuable source of education for many doctors but it has to be remembered that their role is to make profits by encouraging more use of their products. For instance, there are many non-steroidal anti-inflammatory drugs advertised for osteoarthritis but none of these advertisements ever describe their drug as being best reserved for patients who fail to respond to non-pharmacological treatments or to paracetamol. In preventing stroke, the thiazide diuretics are inexpensive and no drug has ever been shown to be superior, yet this is omitted from advertisements of newer, more costly drugs for blood pressure. Finally, advertisements always portray a good outcome and fail to mention the often not insubstantial risk of serious adverse effects. The content of this advertising is therefore often biased

- The key weapon in selling drugs is, however, the pharmaceutical representative who is carefully trained in selling techniques. Not the least of these is giving small presents like pens etc. The point of these gifts is several fold – it creates a desire to reciprocate (by prescribing the representative's product) and it puts a reminder of the name of the product in front of the doctor. The representative is the most expensive part of the industry's portfolio of promotion but also the most powerful – in effect engaging in a 'consultation' with the doctor and having the face-to-face opportunity to negotiate a satisfactory (to the company) endpoint.

- The industry invests heavily in promotion – one estimate from several years ago valued this at £10 000 per doctor per year and it is probably substantially more than this now. The industry might argue that the promotion only encourages the choice of product, i.e. the decision what to prescribe rather than whether to prescribe at all, but this is a direct parallel with the tobacco industry which argued that cigarette advertising might only encourage people to change brand but not to smoke where otherwise they would not. This argument in relation to cigarette advertising is now rejected of course, and it seems reasonable to assume that part of the role of promotion of pharmaceuticals is to encourage prescribing where it would not have otherwise happened. Some of this may be appropriate, e.g. where patients have been undertreated, but some of it is not and may lead to overuse of medicines in places where fewer or even no drugs should be used. A key target for the representatives is the 'innovator', the doctor who wants to try everything new (but who is also fickle and who will drop the drug as soon as something newer comes along). This doctor will help the representative get a foot in the door to win over the more conservative local doctors ('Dr X is prescribing our new drug now, don't you think you should try it too?'). From there, the drug spreads into the 'early adopters', who are slower to take it up but more likely to stick with it, then the 'late adopters' and finally the 'laggards'.

- So does promotion lead to less rational prescribing? It is difficult to study this but it is clear that doctors who prescribe less rationally (i.e. more expensively when lower-cost alternatives were available and with higher rates of prescribing) are more likely to be those who meet with a lot of representatives. However, it is hard to say which is the chicken and which the egg. Does the doctor prescribe more because he sees more representatives or is it the other way around?

- There is an important point here for non-medical prescribers: pharmaceutical companies find it more and more difficult to access doctors, and most doctors, if only by experience, have a some degree of cynicism with regard to the biased messages of the industry. Companies now clearly feel that non-medical prescribers – perhaps nurses more than pharmacists – are a good alternative target for their activities, with responsibilities for prescribing and for influencing colleagues, and perhaps a little naïve. Good advice on how to manage the representatives was provided by the Drugs and Therapeutics Bulletin some years ago (Anon. 1983).

- The NHS: Since most of us want to support the broader aims of the NHS, its efforts to influence our prescribing are particularly powerful psychological and social influences on us to prescribe in certain ways. GPs have prescribing budgets to remind them of the costs of what they prescribe, set by the primary care trusts, and primary care trusts and hospitals are also responsible for the clinical governance of the care they provide, including prescribing. They will therefore try to improve the quality of prescribing while containing costs as much as possible. They will do this in a variety of ways: professionally by education; newsletters; peer support or pressure; and managerially by budget setting; negotiations with hospitals or other providers; and configuring other services (e.g. how many nurse independent prescribers or supplementary prescribers they need and where). There is a range of other NHS resources to support prescribing – these are outlined in other chapters. One of the key aims of these services is to help us to translate the research evidence of how best to treat patients into practice – often a tall order, and outside the remit of this chapter.

Placebos

A placebo (Latin 'I will please') is an inert or inactive substance or a sham procedure knowingly prescribed or undertaken, not for its specific pharmacological or physiological effect, but for its non-specific psychological or psycho-physiological therapeutic effect. The importance of these effects was often underplayed in the past. The development of the randomised controlled trial showed the true power of this effect. For instance, in mild depression, the response to a supposedly therapeutic drug might be 70% (a doctor who prescribed such a drug might feel very satisfied that he can take credit for such a satisfactory outcome) – but the response to a placebo in the same trial can be as high as 60%. This reflects in part the natural history of the condition (most patients get better whatever you do) but also the ability of the placebo to bring about a physical improvement by influencing the patient's expectations and hopes. Some feel that the use of a placebo is unethical, as it is basically lying to a patient (albeit, in a stark example of medical paternalism, for the patient's own good). Nevertheless all doctors recognise the effects of reassurance to a patient, and acknowledging the patient's distress in some way, and all use this placebo effect to some degree. In Britain, there are no legally prescribable placebos, and sometimes patients are prescribed what might be harmless drugs, such as water-soluble vitamins. However, we also use more powerful drugs like antibiotics in this way, and then claim the credit. This has disadvantages: it puts the patient at risk of potentially serious adverse effects, it is fundamentally dishonest and may undermine the prescriber–patient relationship, and it may even lead to us deluding ourselves.

There is also a 'nocebo' (I will harm) effect when an innocuous substance apparently produces adverse effects – this is seen in most clinical trials to some degree where a 'placebo' is used. So these psychological influences can work either way depending on how they are communicated to a patient.

The placebo effect is very important and underestimated. We should use it with caution and as rarely as possible, depending instead on honest reassurance and information to the patient. But there are times when we should use this effect knowingly and without deceiving ourselves.

So why do patients want prescriptions?

This is of course the other side of the coin. Perhaps, to start with, the key question is:

• Do patients actually want a prescription?

Research seems to suggest prescribers tend to overrate the patient's expectation of a prescription (though perhaps not by as much as was previously thought – see below). Indeed the public are often averse to wanting drugs – something that the professionals often overlook. Some patients will refuse prescriptions, either directly or indirectly, by simply not getting the prescription filled or not taking the tablets. Concordance addresses many of these issues.

Patient pressure

Another factor is what doctors perceive as patient pressure for prescriptions. Some doctors believe that patients are never satisfied without a prescription, and act accordingly. Harris categorised this as 'avoidance' because it is in effect an avoidance of the alternative strategy of spending more time with patients to clarify their views and the nature of their problems.

Is there evidence of a great and unreasonable desire for medication from patients? How reasonable is it for doctors to put the blame for the increased volume of prescribing over the past two decades on to 'patient pressure'? Some reject the concept of patient pressure and argue that patients' views are more involved, with beliefs about medicines being more complex than 'wants an antibiotic'.

Britten and co-workers (Britten et al. 2002) conducted semi-structured interviews with 30 adults and later more extensive questionnaires with several hundred adults to reveal their attitudes to medicines. Patients held a variety of views, some of which might be considered 'orthodox' and others 'unorthodox'. The orthodox views held might be considered medically legitimate, and they relate to a positive view of medicines, taken for a broadly biomedical reason, and with a high expectation for a prescription. Other patients held more unorthodox views, in which there were powerful negative views about medicines and their adverse effects, a feeling that at least some doctors over-prescribed and a low desire and expectation for a prescription. The key point was that many patients held both orthodox and unorthodox views simultaneously, and were very ambivalent about their medicines and medicine taking – on the one hand, recognising that the medicines were for their own benefit and, on the other hand, that medicines can cause adverse effects and perhaps wanting to reject the whole sick role. It is little wonder that compliance with medicines is so poor and concordance so difficult to achieve.

When GPs are surveyed, they often describe high levels of demand for prescriptions, but objective evidence consistently suggests that doctors overestimate patients' expectations. Early studies suggested that many patients interviewed in waiting rooms claimed to want advice or reassurance only, at least as often as a prescription. More recent studies in inner city areas suggest that the figure is as high as 67% wanting a prescription – particularly high in patients who were exempt from prescription charges, and older patients. There is evidence that the doctor responds to what they perceive to be patient expectation (whether this is real or not), even when the doctor thinks that a prescription is not strictly medically necessary.

In a study (MacFarlane et al. 1997), 76 GPs recorded clinical data, their certainty about their prescribing decision and any influences on that decision in 1014 consecutive previously well adults suffering with lower respiratory infection. The patients did a similar exercise. Most patients believed that bacterial infection was the problem, antibiotics were the answer and expected a prescription. The doctors thought that antibiotics were not indicated in many of these patients but were often influenced to prescribe, nevertheless, by the patients' expectations. Patients who expected an antibiotic but did not receive one were twice as likely to re-consult as those who did not expect an antibiotic, although their clinical outcomes were no worse.

A key issue here is the quality of the doctor's consultation skills, and how well the doctor negotiates a therapeutic contract with the patient. Longer consultations can reduce prescribing rates but if the consultation goes on too long, prescribing rates increase again as all kinds of hidden agendas/diagnoses start to appear.

We should therefore be working to help prescribers and patients talk to one another more clearly, and this is a key aim of concordance.

Reasons for wanting a prescription

Many reasons and motives have been described. Some of these include:

- The patient perceives therapeutic effect for themselves or others. This is almost a biomedical-type belief in the power of medicines, which may not be in line with the professionals' more scientific beliefs on this point of course. There are also sometimes elements of superstition around the power of the prescription. This is discussed more under 'health beliefs' below.
- To avoid expenditure (e.g. a prescription for Calpol for a child rather than buying it from a pharmacy perhaps?).
- To sanction or make contact with the doctor.
- To achieve recognition of the sick role and to legitimise time off work or school.
- Suggestion by an opinion leader (e.g. mother or friend).
- Because it repeats a previous experience (see below about sore throats as an example of this).
- To receive a 'gift' from the doctor. Many patients end up taking drugs they perhaps didn't really want or need because they don't want to reject the doctor's advice or his or her human response to the patient's distress.
  And so on…

Health beliefs

The health beliefs of patients are determined by many factors, many of which are 'cultural'. Attitudes to medicines seem to vary between nations and even among communities within the same nation. The origins of these beliefs are difficult to establish, but it is clear that many are based in myth and legend, and are centuries old. Others develop within a short time, influenced by public opinion, the media and perhaps by information derived from authoritarian or scientific expert sources. Even the latter beliefs, arising in recent years, are often firmly rooted in myth and image. Is Viagra the answer to unsatisfactory sexual relationships? Is orlistat a solution to obesity?

These influences are passed on by comment on others' personal experience, in jokes, in learned debates, in the media of all types (often with pharmaceutical industry influence), and by one's own experience of what seems to be important, what seems to work and what doesn't. The intangible nature of the whole process stems in part from the fact that for most people, the strongest influences on their own beliefs are the images that are passed on by those near to us. Only rarely will those images be based on any controlled or scientifically evaluated experience. Many of the beliefs become self-fulfilling prophecies, or superstitions, which take an increasingly secure hold despite the weakness of their origins.

An important question arises about the power of experience to influence these beliefs. If an average person is offered an antibiotic for a cold or a sore throat, by a doctor for whom they have respect, what happens to their readiness to seek antibiotics in the future? Will they dismiss the experience as perhaps not fitting in with what they have learned from other doctors in the rest of their lifetime, or will they change their views because of that act, and because no great adversity has affected them subsequently?

Such an experiment was performed in Southampton (Little et al. 1997). The original idea of the study was to perform a randomised controlled trial to see if the strategy of giving antibiotics for a sore throat only when it was essential as defined by very firm medical criteria, or a more liberal attitude to routine use of antibiotics for sore throats, regularly made an important clinical difference to outcomes (it didn't). But what was noticed was that the patients who received the antibiotics were, as a group, more likely to return for antibiotics if they suffered a further episode of sore throat, and they were more positively oriented towards antibiotics than those who never received them, even though at the end of the day these patients were no better for having received the antibiotics. These patients had been 'taught' that antibiotics were the appropriate response to a sore throat.

Race and culture

Some health beliefs go deeper and seem to be engrained in some specific cultures. In prescribing, it is important to have some understanding of transcultural issues and how these will affect how patients view the prescription and the need for a medicine. Some ethnic minorities tend to have fixed views about this. In some cultures, disease is seen as always something external to the patient and must therefore be fought off with external aid, such as a prescription medicine. In some ethnic minorities, a mother who did not bring her child to the doctor at the first sign of an infection would be considered a bad parent. By follow on, a doctor who does not prescribe (and legitimise the whole process) may lose contact with the family, who may avoid that doctor in the future. These pressures can be subtle and require an awareness and sensitivity on the part of the prescriber. Sometimes they are less subtle – a GP might lose a large proportion of his patients and hence affect his income if he tries to impose a very different attitude concerning prescribing to that of his patients. One often has to move slowly in these matters.

For example, a study in London in the 1990s (Morgan 1995) examined the attitudes of white and Afro-Caribbean patients with hypertension to their medicines and medicine taking. The white patients were more likely than the Afro-Caribbeans to take their medicines as prescribed, and tended to have better blood pressure control as a result. The Afro-Caribbean patients often had traditional cultural beliefs about long-term harmful effects of drugs and often sought an alternative resource in terms of herbal remedies. There was a cultural gulf and lack of communication between Afro-Caribbean patients and their GPs who did not appreciate these issues.

But even within what might seem to be a homogeneous culture, there can be wide variations in subcultures. For instance, within white British populations, attitudes to medicines will vary from the well-heeled *Sunday Times* reader who wants to discuss a range of therapeutic options for a problem, including complementary treatments, to the older more stoical patient who does not want to trouble the doctor, to other patients who want medicines (any medicines!) for every little ailment.

The key point is that one should not stereotype patients and that every patient is different, and deserves and needs to have their own needs and beliefs explored if the prescriber is to help the patient properly.

Patients and the media

Increasingly the media influence us all in our day-to-day habits, in the food we eat, in the presents we purchase for Christmas and birthdays, and perhaps even in the medicines we swallow. The media portrays sensation and tends to see medicines either as 'wonder' drugs or as 'killer' drugs: the notion that what is a wonder drug in one situation can also be a killer in another is a subtlety that banner headlines cannot deal with. In recent years, the media coverage for some new drugs has been intense, for instance, with sildenafil (Viagra) – perhaps a potent mix of sex, money and science! This has certainly raised public awareness of the drug, which may be good if it allows some patients with conditions which can be helped by sildenafil to overcome their reticence and come forward, but which may be harmful if it encourages the use of this drug for normal men who feel that their sexual prowess could be enhanced further. There has been little in the media about the potential adverse medical effects of this drug. It is less clear what the actual effects of media coverage have been, in terms of encouraging drug sales. Nevertheless, newspapers and television can greatly increase awareness of a drug and its use when this has a very weak scientific basis.

Another example might be the uptake of vaccinations with MMR, which has fallen drastically after adverse publicity that it might be associated with autism or inflammatory bowel disease. Statements by various scientific bodies have not been able to redress the powerful negative perceptions in some parts of the general public and as a result there is now a real risk of an epidemic of these possibly serious childhood illnesses. While the scientific evidence is soundly in favour of immunisation, the public have had doubts instilled in their minds by the constant media hype, creating uncertainty. The positive images of the unbounded benefits of science of the 1950s and 1960s has given way to a much more guarded view of science, largely as a result of many problems and disasters ranging from thalidomide to pollution. The social group most influenced against immunisation are the middle classes, perhaps reflecting better education in some areas (but not often in science).

In Europe, companies are not allowed advertise their prescription-only drugs to the general public, but are allowed to advertise over-the-counter medicines generally. Despite this ban, there is a steady business in the media of almost 'advertorials' in newspapers and magazines that effectively promote particular prescription-only drugs. In countries where direct advertising of prescription medicines is allowed, such as New Zealand or the United States, there have been many concerns about the harmful effects of encouraging patients to seek perhaps inappropriate drugs. In the United States, many drugs are openly advertised on the internet, where there is a plethora of information available – some good, some appallingly poor. This is all increasingly accessible to patients everywhere, so there may seem to be plenty of information available – in reality such an information overload can often result in patients ending up more poorly informed about their drugs as a result of misinformation.

There is a dilemma here: the professionals might like the public's access to such information restricted since it might actually harm patients (but also might diminish their professional power); on the other hand, this information might benefit patients who are not receiving the medicines they should, or who can learn more about the medicines they are taking. The key concern here should be access to unbiassed information, which we should encourage, but which is sadly not often available. Healthcare professionals have to help patients through this morass.

So the media can be a powerful influence with both advantages and disadvantages, and one that is likely to persist.

Conclusions

We have briefly examined a wide range of psychological and sociological influences on prescribing that act either directly on doctors or on patients (and hence indirectly on the doctors). There is little information or study so far of non-medical prescribers but it is very likely that all of the influences we have listed (and many we have not) will also affect nurses, pharmacists and others in the same way. They may be even more influential in the short term in nurses and pharmacists, since dealing with these influences is part of medical culture handed down from trainer to trainee – this experience dose not exist yet with other professions. These issues will be of great importance in helping patients to use their medicines properly and in achieving concordance with them about the aims and details of their treatment.

There are two key areas of skills to be learnt to remedy any potential harmful effect of these influences:

- The first is self-reflection: to be aware of these influences and to recognise them when they occur; to be able to reflect on one's own prescribing and consider how influential these are on you as a prescriber; and to compare your prescribing and behaviour in this respect to that of your peers, or better still to some professional ideal. Then you can decide whether you have struck the proper balance.

- The second key skills are those of the consultation, where good communication (listening to the patient and understanding their point of view, as well as getting yours across to them) and an ability to negotiate (being prepared to trade, agree compromise and sell the deal) are essential.

References

Anon. (1983). Getting good value from drug reps. *Drugs and Therapeutics Bulletin 21*(4): 13–15.

Bradley, C.P. (1991). Decision making and prescribing patterns – a literature review. *Family Practice 8*: 276–287.

Britten, N., Ukoumunne, O.C., Boulton, M.G. (2002). Patients' attitudes to medicines and expectations for prescriptions. *Health Expect-ations 5*: 256–269.

Gilbert, D., Walley, T., New, B. (2000). Lifestyle medicines. *British Medical Journal 321*: 1341–1344.

Harris, C.M., Heywood, P.L., Clayden, A.D. (1990). *The Analysis of Prescribing in General Practice: a Guide to Audit and Research*. London: HMSO.

Howie, J.G. (1976). Clinical judgement and antibiotic use in general practice. *British Medical Journal 2*: 1061–1064.

Illich, I. (1981). *Medical Nemesis.* London: Penguin.

Little, P., Gould, C., Williamson, I., et al. (1997). Reattendance and complications in a randomised trial of prescribing strategies for sore throat: the medicalising effect of prescribing antibiotics. *British Medical Journal 315*: 350–352.

Macfarlane, J., Holmes, W., Macfarlane, R., et al. (1997). Influence of patients' expectations on antibiotic management of acute lower respiratory tract illness in general practice: questionnaire study. *British Medical Journal 315*: 1211–1214.

Morgan, M. (1995). The significance of ethnicity for health promotion – patients' use of anti-hypertensive drugs in inner London. *International Journal Of Epidemiology 24* Suppl 1: S79–S84.

Applied pharmacology

Michele Cossey

Clinical pharmacology is defined as the application of scientific principles to understanding the ways in which drugs behave and work in humans (Weatherall et al. 2006).

A good general understanding of basic pharmacology and how it is applied to the treatment of patients is essential for any prescriber. It is not enough to have knowledge of how an individual drug may exert its effect. A prescriber must also understand how differences in individuals and populations may alter this effect. This understanding will allow prescribers to make decisions about routes of administration, dosing, frequency of administration, contraindications, adverse effects and interactions with other drugs. In order to be able to prescribe appropriately and effectively, prescribers need to appreciate the concepts of how the body handles drugs, i.e. *pharmacokinetics* and how these may be altered or influenced and, once in the body, how drugs can exert their effect and what may alter this potential effect, i.e. *pharmacodynamics*.

This chapter covers the essential elements of basic applied pharmacology. It will aim to give readers an overview of the general concepts of both pharmacokinetics and pharmacodynamics and how these influence drug choice, dose and effect. It will also briefly cover adverse drug reactions and interactions, how these may occur and what the prescriber can do to minimise these where possible. Finally, it will bring the knowledge of these concepts together in order to provide a practical framework for individualising drug therapy.

In a chapter of this length, it is only possible to give a basic overview. A more in-depth review of this subject can be found in the references and further reading provided at the end of this chapter.

Pharmacokinetic principles

Pharmacokinetics can simplistically be described as how the body handles drugs over a period of time. It is a complex subject but a general understanding of the basic principles is essential for good prescribing practice. The basic principles that a prescriber needs knowledge of are absorption, distribution, metabolism and excretion (ADME), together with the route and dose of drug administered. The general principles of ADME can be summarised in Figure 7.1. These will be explained further in the following sections.

Routes of administration

Drugs may act locally or systemically. Locally implies that the effects of the drug are confined to a specific area. Systemically means that a drug has to enter the circulation in order to be delivered to its site of action. Drugs may be administered to a patient in a number of different ways, for example, via the mouth (orally), via the skin (transdermally), via a mucous membrane (sublingual tablets or spray) or via the injectable route (parenteral administration). The

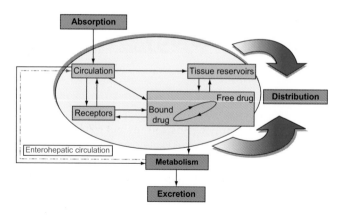

Figure 7.1 The general principles of ADME

method of delivery into the body will influence the amount of drug reaching the circulation, the intended site of action and ultimately, the effect of that drug.

The term *bioavailability* is used to explain what proportion of an administered dose of drug will reach the circulation unaltered and therefore able to have an effect. Bioavailability (F) is a factor of the *extent* of drug absorption, not the *rate* of drug absorption. The amount of drug reaching the systemic circulation can be calculated if you know the bioavailability and the dose administered.

Amount of drug reaching the systemic circulation = F x dose

Some drugs have different bioavailability properties for different formulations and therefore dosing alterations may be needed when changing between formulations, for example, when switching patients from phenytoin capsules or tablets to phenytoin suspension.

A drug given by intravenous (IV) injection will have a bioavailability of 1.0 as 100% of the dose is administered directly into the circulation. A drug given by the oral route will have a reduced bioavailability due the effects of ADME. The chosen route of administration will depend on many factors including the condition to be treated, the required onset of drug action, patient preference and available methods of delivery. The aim of the prescriber is to select the most appropriate route of administration that will be both clinically effective and cost effective. For example, in the treatment of asthma, drug therapy is delivered by inhaler directly into the lungs where the effect is required, while in the case of eczema, drug therapy may be applied directly to the affected area. The prescriber must make an initial decision based on the clinical condition requiring treatment, the available routes of administration, the absorption characteristics of the drug formulation and the required site of action.

Absorption

Almost all drugs, other than those, for example, administered by IV injection, must be absorbed before they can exert their effect. Drugs that exert their effect systemically must cross at least one cell in order to reach the circulation. Most drugs do this by passive diffusion (i.e. movement from an area of high concentration to an area of low concentration), for example, in crossing through the wall of the small intestine, where there is high concentration, into the bloodstream, where there is low concentration. However, some drugs, e.g. levadopa and fluorouracil, require special transport mechanisms in order to cross cell membranes. These 'active transport' mechanisms are not very important in terms of drug absorption but are essential in ensuring maintenance of cellular function by transport of ions, e.g. potassium, sugars and amino acids, across cell walls.

The rate and extent of drug absorption across a cell membrane will be determined by a number of factors.

Lipid solubility

The lipid solubility of a drug will determine how easily it will pass across a cell membrane. Cell membranes are composed of a double layer of phospholipids and so lipid soluble drugs (or lipophilic drugs) will pass though cell membranes more easily than water soluble drugs. Therefore, the more lipid soluble a drug, the easier it is for that drug to be absorbed from the small intestine after oral administration. This fact is used in the design and manufacture of drugs. For example, if a manufacturer wanted to formulate a drug to act directly within the gut, e.g. for Crohn's disease, they would look to develop a more water soluble (or low lipid soluble) drug, so that the drug is held within the gut and not absorbed from the small intestine. Another determination is the state of ionisation (i.e. whether the drug carries a positive or negative charge and to what extent; or whether it carries no charge and is considered neutral) of a drug, as only un-ionised drug is lipid soluble.

Surface area for absorption

The larger the surface area available for absorption, the quicker the process will occur. The small intestine is designed to provide a very large surface area for drug absorption to take place, due to a large number of villi and a very rich blood supply. If a patient has a condition that reduces the potential area for drug absorption, e.g. inflammatory bowel disease, then the relative absorption of a drug will be reduced, thus interfering with the amount of drug available in the circulation and ultimately the effect of that drug.

Gastric motility and emptying

Most absorption takes place in the small intestine. This means that drugs taken orally need to be disintegrated in the stomach and delivered via emptying of the gastric contents into the intestine. Therefore, anything that alters gastric motility and emptying will result in altering the rate of absorption.

The presence of food after a meal will slow gastric emptying. If drugs are taken with food, then their absorption and clinical effect may be delayed. This is why generally it is important to ensure that drugs are prescribed to be taken either before or some time after a meal. This ensures quicker delivery to the site of absorption and prevents delaying the drug effect. Counselling the patient on when to take their drugs is therefore very important.

Sometimes drugs are prescribed to be taken with food. This is to lessen side effects by preventing large concentrations from entering the circulation so that the drug is absorbed in a steadier manner, due to slower gastric emptying. It is also to prevent local side effects, like irritation of the stomach lining, by using the food as a barrier, for example, when prescribing non-steroidal anti-inflammatory drugs (NSAIDs).

Some illnesses or conditions may affect gastric motility and therefore drug absorption. Gastric emptying may be slowed during a migraine attack and therefore oral analgesics may not act quickly enough. This can be addressed by giving the drug via another route, e.g. subcutaneous injection, or by combining the oral analgesic with a drug to speed up gastric motility, e.g. metoclopramide.

However, the whole process of gastric motility and emptying and its effect on drug absorption is very complex. In some cases, delayed gastric emptying may actually be beneficial to drug absorption. For example, some drugs, such as nitrofurantoin, may be better dissolved or disintegrated as a result of spending longer in the stomach's acidic environment.

The prescriber should check what instructions a patient may require regarding taking drugs with food and patients should be fully counselled on all their medication.

First pass metabolism

Some drugs when given orally are absorbed from the small intestine directly into the hepatic portal vein and are transported directly to the liver. As the liver is the main organ for metabolism, these drugs are then metabolised either partially or fully by the liver. This means that the amount of drug entering the circulation is either reduced or completely negated. This effect is known as 'first pass metabolism'. Some drugs, e.g. glyceryl trinitrate, when swallowed are almost totally inactivated via the first pass metabolism effect and are therefore administered by another route. (In the case of glyceryl trinitrate, by sublingual spray or tablet.) Other drugs may still be active even after first pass metabolism if their metabolites are active, e.g. propranolol metabolised to the active 4-hydroxypropranolol. In practical terms, prescribers can often assume that a drug has been formulated to take account of any first pass metabolism effect and therefore rarely have to consider it.

Time

The amount of time that a drug is in contact with the walls of the small intestine will affect its absorption. Anything that alters gut transit time, e.g. gastroenteritis, will affect time for absorption. Conversely, hypomotility of the gastrointestinal tract may result in higher concentrations of drug entering the circulation.

Blood flow

Depending on how drugs are administered, the blood flow to the site of administration will affect the rate of absorption. Blood flow to the gut is usually high and this allows for good absorption into the circulation. Some areas of the body have variable blood flow, e.g. muscles, and so absorption from intra-muscular injection may vary, depending on other physical aspects of the patient which may require muscle blood flow to be increased or decreased.

As described above, there are a number of factors that will influence the absorption of a drug from its site of action into the circulation. Prescribers need to understand how the factors discussed above may affect drug absorption and how they can be used to ensure drug dosing is appropriate and formulation choices are rational in order to ensure effective absorption and delivery of the drug to its site of action.

Distribution

Once a drug is absorbed from its site of administration into the circulation, it is transported around the body to its site of action. This process is known as distribution. Unless a drug reaches its site of action in an adequate concentration, it will not be able to exert its effect. As with absorption, there are factors that will influence the distribution of drugs around the body.

Blood flow

The rate and extent to which organs and tissues are perfused with blood will directly affect the distribution of drug to those areas. This, in turn, will affect the rate and extent of drug action at that site. Organs and tissues that receive high blood perfusion, e.g. heart, kidneys and brain, will rapidly receive a drug and have a much greater potential to receive an adequate concentration for the drug to have an effect. Poorly perfused organs and tissues, e.g. fat, muscle and bone, may take some time to receive adequate concentrations.

Protein binding

Most drugs that enter the circulation are poorly soluble. This means that in order to move around the body via the circulatory system, some proportion of the drug needs to be 'carried'. These 'carriers' are generally plasma proteins and drug molecules are either 'free' in the circulation or 'bound' to these proteins. It should be noted that only free drug can cross plasma membranes (as drugs bound to plasma proteins are large) and therefore can exert an effect. This state of plasma binding is a reversible process. A drug may enter the circulation and be partially or wholly bound to plasma proteins but over time the drug is released from this protein binding site or free drug may bind to plasma proteins. This is a dynamic process that allows for equilibrium to be reached between the fraction of bound and unbound (free) drug.

Albumin is the most abundant plasma protein and generally drugs that are acidic in nature bind to albumin, while drugs that are alkali in nature bind to α_1-acid glycoprotein. The process of drug binding to plasma protein is a competitive one. This means that if more than one drug that binds to plasma protein is present at the same time in the circulation, these drugs will compete for the plasma protein binding sites.

This is an important concept to understand, particularly for drugs that are highly protein-bound and have a narrow *therapeutic index*, e.g. warfarin. A narrow therapeutic index means that the concentration of drug needed to have therapeutic effect is very close to that which may be either toxic or ineffective. This is shown in Figure 7.2.

In most cases small alterations in protein binding should not have a significant clinical effect. However, in some patients who may be on multiple drug treatments, the potential for drug interactions is increased. This may become clinically important if one drug displaces another drug from its protein binding sites due to competition for these sites. This can be shown in the following example.

Drug W is highly protein-bound (90%). Therefore if the patient is prescribed 100 mg we can assume that 90 mg (90%) is protein-bound and the remaining 10 mg (10%) is free drug. As described earlier, free drug is therapeutically active. If the patient is also prescribed other

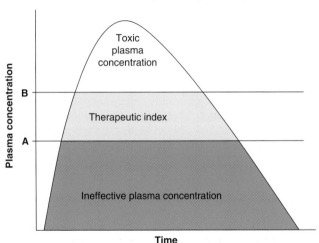

Figure 7.2 Diagrammatic representation of therapeutic index

drugs which compete for protein binding sites and these drugs displace drug W from some of its binding sites then protein binding for drug W will decrease. If drug W is displaced then the amount of unbound (or free drug) will increase.

If we use our 100 mg dose and assume that drug W is now only 85% protein-bound (due to displacement from its binding sites), this means that 85 mg is now bound and 15 mg is unbound (or free). This is only a small change of 5 mg in terms of free drug (from 10 mg to 15 mg). However, the actual percentage change in free drug can be shown to be 50% by the following equation:

$$\frac{5\,\text{mg change in free drug}}{100} = x\,(\%\,\text{change})\times 10\,\text{mg}$$

where x = 50%.

A 50% change in unbound (free) drug could be clinically important, particularly if the drug has a narrow therapeutic index or if there are any problems with metabolism or excretion, for example, reduced renal or hepatic function

If in this example drug W is warfarin (which is highly protein-bound) and it is competing with other drugs for binding sites, more warfarin may be displaced from these binding sites and will remain free in the circulation. This free drug can be metabolised and excreted. However a 50% increase in unbound, active warfarin may cause the patient to bleed due to the higher plasma concentration exerting a potentially greater effect. Tolbutamide is an example of a drug which competes with and can displace warfarin from its binding sites.

Interactions of this type are more likely to be clinically important in the acute setting, for example, in administering loading doses of warfarin before a steady state is reached. Once a drug has reached its steady state then small amounts being displaced from protein binding sites will have less significant effects as metabolism and excretion will deal with these. This is one of the reasons why patients taking warfarin have their International Normalised Ratio (INR), a measure of the blood's clotting time, checked regularly and this monitoring is increased when patients are started on other drugs known to interact with warfarin until they are stabilised on the new combination.

This situation may also arise if a patient is suffering from a disease that alters plasma proteins. For example, a patient with chronic cirrhosis of the liver may have reduced albumin (as this is made by the liver). This means that more of the drug will be free in the circulation than expected and again, the warfarin dose administered may have an increased effect. For this reason, drug doses may be reduced, patients taking warfarin are counselled and their plasma drug concentration is regularly monitored. Figure 7.3 shows the potential impact of altered protein binding on plasma drug concentration.

It is important for the prescriber to understand the concept of protein binding in order to make a decision about drug dosing. In patients with significantly reduced hepatic function or diseases that impact on plasma protein concentrations, drug doses of highly protein-bound drugs should be reduced. The *British National Formulary* (BNF 2009) gives advice on this.

Distribution barriers

For a drug to have an effect, it must reach the tissues. Drugs can access and accumulate in certain tissues and cannot gain access to other tissues, due to the existence of barriers. The blood–brain barrier is made up of different endothelial cells that only allow highly lipid soluble drugs to cross over into the brain tissue. A drug that is poorly lipid soluble will have great difficulty in crossing this barrier and will have little or no effect on the brain. However, an anaesthetic agent, which is

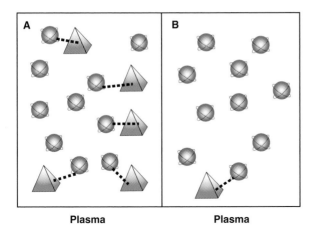

Figure 7.3 The potential impact of altered protein binding on plasma drug concentration

In **A** there is an equilibrium between free drug ⊗ and drug bound to plasma proteins ◭⋯⊗

In **B** as the concentration of the plasma protein ◭ falls (for example, in liver disease) the concentration of free drug X increases.

As free drug is active there is more drug available to target receptors and have an increased effect.

formulated to be highly lipid soluble, will pass through this barrier. While some of the anaesthetic may pass into other tissues (e.g. muscle or fat stores), the vast majority of the drug will cross the blood–brain barrier and as the brain has a higher blood perfusion than that of muscle or fat, the drug will have the desired effect of rapid anaesthesia.

In pregnancy, the placenta forms a barrier between the mother's circulation and that of the foetus. Some drugs which are highly lipophilic can cross this barrier, e.g. morphine and ethanol, while other poorly lipid soluble molecules cannot easily pass through. Prescribing and drug dosing in pregnancy is a very specialist area and prescribers should always seek specialist advice before making decisions about prescribing for pregnant women.

Volume of distribution

When a drug is given and enters the circulation, it may bind to plasma proteins (as described above) in order to be carried and distributed around the body. Once in the general circulation, the drug can exert its effect by binding to specific receptor sites or it may bind to other tissues where it has no pharmacological effect, for example, fat tissue or certain organs. The term *volume of distribution* (Vd) can describe the extent to which a drug is distributed throughout the body and bound to other tissues.

In clinical practice we can estimate the volume of distribution if we know the dose the patient received and a measured plasma concentration at a given time. This estimate is referred to as the *apparent volume of distribution* and provides us with a theoretical volume of fluid needed to dilute a known dose of drug to produce the measured plasma concentration.

For example, if a patient is administered a 100 mg intravenous bolus dose and the measured plasma concentration is 10 mg/L, the apparent volume of distribution can be estimated to be 10 L. However if the plasma concentration was measured to be 1 mg/L, the corresponding volume of distribution would be estimated to be much larger at 100 L.

- When a drug has a *low* apparent volume of distribution, this suggests it is confined mainly to the bloodstream and body water.
- When a drug has a *high* apparent volume of distribution, this suggests it is distributed widely to other tissues.

An understanding of this concept may be useful in drug overdose where, for example, haemodialysis is used to try to clear the drug from the circulation. If most of the drug is distributed and bound to other tissues, i.e. the volume of distribution is high and little of the drug is actually present in the circulation, then haemodialysis may be ineffective. Volume of distribution can also be affected by a patient's weight, body water content or fat distribution.

In practical terms, the prescriber can assume that the volume of distribution of a drug has been taken into account during the formulation of that drug. A more in-depth view of the volume of distribution can be found in some of the further reading at the end of this chapter.

Once a drug is in the circulation and distributed around the body, in order to have its effect, the body must have mechanisms in place to excrete the drug. In order to effectively excrete drugs from the body, they are first metabolised.

Metabolism

Drug metabolism or biotransformation is the process of modifying or altering the chemical composition of the drug. As described previously, the more lipid soluble and unionised a drug, the more easily it passes across cell membranes. It would seem logical then, that in order to remove the pharmacological activity and actively excrete a drug, the body should attempt to make the drug more water soluble (hydrophilic) and less lipid soluble, as well as making the drug more polar (or ionised). This means that when a drug enters the kidney for excretion, it is unlikely to be reabsorbed across the cell membranes back into the general circulation.

Most drug metabolism occurs in the liver where a series of enzymes catalyse numerous biochemical reactions. These reactions can be classified into two phases, *Phase 1* and *Phase 2*. Some drugs may undergo both Phase 1 and Phase 2 metabolism, some may only undergo only one of these phases and some may undergo Phase 2 before Phase 1. There are also some drugs that are excreted unchanged, without being actively metabolised.

Phase 1

The process of Phase 1 metabolism results in oxidation, reduction or hydrolysis of a drug. The process of oxidation is the most common and often catalysed by one of the many cytochrome P450 isoenzymes (CYP450). Although the aim of this process is to render the drug less effective and more water soluble, some drugs are actually made pharmacologically active by this process. For example, enalapril is pharmacologically inactive, but its Phase 1 metabolite enalaprilat is active. In some cases, the resulting metabolite of an active drug is itself pharmacologically active, e.g. diamorphine metabolised to morphine.

Phase 2

Drugs or Phase 1 metabolites that are not sufficiently polar, or are still active, are made more hydrophilic by the process of conjugation. This process involves the drug or metabolite being attached to an endogenous compound, for example, a glucuronate. The resulting compounds are more readily excreted by the kidneys, as they are more water soluble and polar in nature. As with Phase 1, some drugs are still active after conjugation, e.g. morphine is metabolised to morphine-6-glucuronide, which still exerts an analgesic effect.

Cytochrome P450 iso-enzymes

Before leaving drug metabolism, it is necessary to take a closer look at the CYP450 enzyme group and how affecting these enzymes can have major effects on the excretion of certain drugs.

Some drugs can increase the rate of synthesis and action of CYP450 enzymes and are known as enzyme inducers, e.g. rifampicin, while other drugs can inhibit this process and are known as drug inhibitors, e.g. cimetidine (Table 7.1 gives some examples of clinically important inducers and inhibitors). Generally, induction requires that the CYP450 enzymes are exposed to the enzyme inducer for some time, while enzyme inhibitors can exert their effect on the CYP450 system soon after exposure.

Sometimes, it is not just drugs that can affect this CYP450 system. Exogenous substances can also affect it and if these substances are taken at the same time as drug therapy, then they can affect the action of the drug. A good example of this is grapefruit juice, which is known to inhibit the CYP450 system. Patients taking drugs where plasma concentration is crucial due to a narrow therapeutic index, e.g. theophylline or cyclosporin, are advised not to drink grapefruit juice, as it can slow down the enzyme system and result in a much increased plasma concentration and therapeutic effect of the drug.

A full list of enzyme inducers and inhibitors can be found in the *British National Formulary* (BNF 2009). A more in-depth review of the effect of fruit juices on liver enzymes is provided in the further reading at the end of this chapter.

Most drugs are metabolised by concentration-independent mechanisms, i.e. the enzyme responsible for their metabolism is not saturated while the drug is within the therapeutic range. There are some enzymes that can be saturated even when the drug is within this therapeutic range. As this happens, small additional doses can lead to a disproportionate rise in plasma concentration and ultimately to toxicity. An example of this is the drug phenytoin (an antiepileptic). This drug has a narrow therapeutic index and the enzyme responsible for its metabolism becomes saturated within its therapeutic range, so small increases in dose can cause increases in plasma concentrations above the therapeutic level and result in toxicity. As there is great inter-patient variability in this response, phenytoin requires careful dosing and plasma monitoring until a patient is stable.

As discussed, the processes of drug metabolism are aimed at making a drug more readily excreted.

Excretion

Most drugs are excreted via the kidney either unchanged or after the processes of metabolism. As described above, the process of drug metabolism may result in a pharmacologically active

Table 7.1. Some examples of methods of administering drugs to patients

Method of administration	Examples of dose form
Oral administration (via the mouth)	Tablets, capsules, solutions, elixirs, suspensions
Topical (via the skin or mucous membranes)	Creams, ointments, gels, lotions, patches (e.g. fentanyl patches, HRT), sprays (e.g. GTN), sublingual preparations
Parenteral (injected or infused **but not** via GI tract), e.g. via intravenous injections, subcutaneous, intramuscular, intrathecal routes	Suitable solution(s) in the appropriate form for administration via chosen route, e.g. oily solution, lipid-based solution etc. Dose forms are generally prepared as sterile preparations for administration via these routes

compound and therefore the effect of the drug will mainly be dependant on excretion, rather than its metabolism.

Renal excretion

The kidneys are very well perfused, receiving approximately 1.5 L per minute of blood. A proportion of this (between 10–20%) is actively filtered by the glomerulus, producing glomerular filtrate. Some drugs or metabolites can pass directly into the kidney at this stage, but they have to be small and therefore drugs or metabolites bound to plasma proteins cannot pass into the kidney in this way, but unbound or free drugs can.

Some drugs are actively secreted from the capillaries into the proximal convoluted tubule of the nephron. This process of tubular secretion is an active process requiring carrier systems and, usually, involves those drugs or metabolites that are strongly acidic or alkali in nature. An example of a drug excreted in this way is penicillin. As this process is an active one, it can be inhibited by, for example, the drug probenecid, which inhibits the active transport mechanism and therefore the excretion of penicillin, thereby increasing the plasma concentration of penicillin.

Some drugs are actively reabsorbed back into the circulation. Active reabsorption enables the body to hold onto vital nutrients and vitamins. Drugs which are still lipid soluble and unionised at urine pH can be reabsorbed during this process and continue to exert their effect. Excretion of these drugs can be influenced by altering the pH of urine, e.g. by administering sodium bicarbonate.

Enterohepatic cycling

Other mechanisms of drug excretion include via the liver, in bile. Once secreted by the liver into bile, they enter the duodenum via the common bile duct and continue on towards the small intestine. Here, some drugs can be deconjugated by the action of gut bacteria and reabsorbed back into the blood stream from the terminal ileum. They then return to the liver by the enterohepatic circulation. The drugs undergo further metabolism and are secreted back into bile and continue going around this process called *enterohepatic cycling*.

This is an important mechanism to understand because although not many drugs are excreted in bile, those that are and that undergo this cycling mechanism can have their effect in the body extended, but also anything that interferes with this mechanism can alter the effect of the drug. For example, the oral contraceptive pill contains oestrogens that are recycled around the body by this mechanism. If a woman is given a course of broad-spectrum antibiotics, these could alter the gut bacteria and therefore, metabolites are not broken down in the small intestine. The oestrogen conjugate is excreted in faeces and enterohepatic cycling is prevented. This can reduce the effect of the oral contraceptive pill. Similarly, diarrhoea can limit the time available for this cycling and also reduce the effect of the pill. Figure 7.4 shows the enterohepatic circulation.

Other methods of excretion

Other methods of excretion include via sweat, breath, tears, saliva and breast milk. These are passive processes and tend to be less important except, of course, when prescribing for nursing mothers. A list of drugs that are excreted in breast milk and the potential consequences is available in the *British National Formulary* (BNF 2009).

Half-life

The term *half-life* ($t_{1/2}$) of a drug is used to describe the time it takes for the plasma concentration to fall to half its original value and is measured in hours. The half-life is the same at all concentrations, i.e. it is a constant factor. Figure 7.5 shows this graphically.

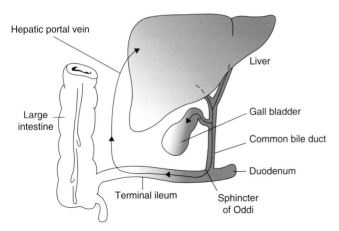

Figure 7.4 The enterohepatic circulation

Hepatic portal vein

Liver

Large intestine

Gall bladder

Common bile duct

Duodenum

Terminal ileum

Sphincter of Oddi

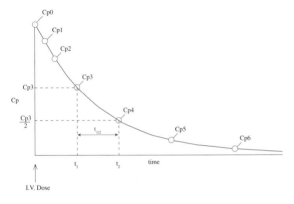

Figure 7.5 Plasma concentration VS time plot for I.V. injection showing how to calculate the half-life ($t_{1/2}$)

When a drug is given in repeated doses, there will come a point when the drug begins to accumulate and a state arises where elimination of the drug by the body matches that being given by the administered dose. This is termed 'steady state'. Drugs with short half-lives reach steady state quicker than those with long half-lives. In order to reach steady state with a drug that has a long half-life, a loading dose may be needed to achieve a therapeutic plasma concentration and this is then followed by smaller maintenance doses, to maintain this plasma concentration or steady state.

Having dealt with the key principles of absorption, distribution, metabolism and excretion (ADME), the prescriber can use this understanding to make some assessments of drug dosing. By using the information already described in this chapter, a prescriber should be able to consider the following points. When a drug is administered, the route of administration determines how quickly it will have its effect. The amount of drug in the circulation and its potential effect will depend on how much is administered, whether the drug is plasma protein-bound or free (i.e. how it is distributed around the body), and how quickly it is metabolised and excreted. The speed at which a drug is excreted by the body is a key factor in determining the duration of action of a drug.

These are the basic principles of pharmacokinetics.

Pharmacodynamics

In the first section, we dealt with how the body deals with drugs, or pharmacokinetics. Pharmacodynamics studies the effects that the drug will have on the body, at both receptor level and on the body's systems as a whole.

The many and varied physiological systems and mechanisms that control all bodily functions are very complex. These functions are kept in check by a myriad of different electrical and chemical messenger systems that work together to maintain the body's homeostatic state. There are many different ways in which the body controls its systems by signalling from one to another in order to switch systems on, off or alter their rate. The body's own endogenous signals that act on receptors are often called *ligands*. The body could not function as it does without the presence of these natural ligands. For example, insulin, noradrenalin and serotonin are all naturally occurring chemical substances within the body which exert their effects by acting as ligands at receptor sites. The body's many types of signalling are too varied and complex to review in detail in this chapter but in-depth reviews of this subject can be found in the further reading.

Drugs exert their effect by altering to one degree or another the body's own physiological systems. In this way drugs act as exogenous ligands. Drugs can act at receptors, at enzyme systems, at ion channels or at carrier mechanisms.

Drugs acting at receptors

Drugs have their effect at receptors by mimicking an endogenous (natural) ligand and binding to a receptor site in the same manner that one of the body's own signalling molecules might do, to form a *ligand-receptor complex*. The receptor sites are usually protein molecules either on the surface of a cell or located intracellularly in the cytoplasm. Obviously drugs act in many different ways and this is because not all drugs can bind to all receptors. In order for a drug to act as a ligand at a particular receptor site it must have a complementary structure to that site. This can be considered in the same way as jigsaw pieces fitting together (Figure 7.6).

The effect of the ligand-receptor complex will vary depending on how the drug exerts its effect. In some cases this drug-ligand complex causes a specific response and these types of ligands are called *agonists*. An example of a drug acting as an agonist is salbutamol, a β_2-receptor agonist used in asthma, which binds to receptors on the smooth muscle in the bronchioles causing bronchodilation. Some ligand-drug complexes do not have an effect but they stop or block a particular natural messenger system from having its effect, and this type of ligand is called an ***antagonist***. An example of a drug acting as an antagonist is atenolol, a β_1-adrenoceptor antagonist used in angina. It is used to block the β_1 effects of noradrenaline on the heart, causing a slowing of the force of contraction, reduction in cardiac oxygen consumption and alleviation of angina pain.

Drug dose–response, agonists and antagonists

Drugs are given to exert a desired effect. Each drug will have a maximal attainable response, which is dependant on the concentration of the drug in the body. The maximum drug response is termed E_{max} and is the maximal effect high concentrations when all available receptors are occupied by the drug. The concentration required to produce half this maximal effect is termed the EC_{50}. This can be shown graphically in Figure 7.7 using a concentration VS effect plot.

Agonists can be described as either *complete* or *partial agonists*. A drug is a complete agonist if it can exert its maximal effect when all receptors are occupied. If it can only exert a submaximal effect (i.e. less than the body's own natural agonist effect) when all receptors are occupied, it is termed a partial agonist. The term *efficacy* is used to describe the ability of a drug to exert an effect at a receptor site. The term *affinity* is used to describe the extent to which a drug binds to a receptor. The greater affinity a drug has for a receptor, the greater the binding between the drug and its chosen receptor will be. Some drugs have greater or lesser affinity for their receptors than others. While drugs may exert an effect at a receptor, the extent of this

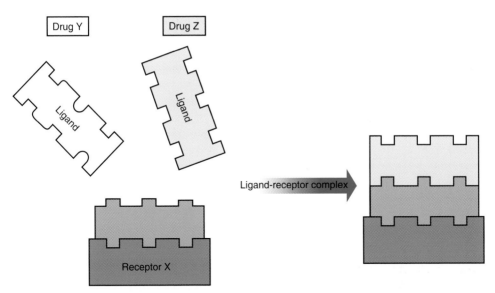

Figure 7.6 Drug-receptor binding. Drug Y cannot bind to receptor X as it is the wrong shape, whereas drug Z has a complementary structure and can therefore bind to receptor X to form a ligand-receptor complex

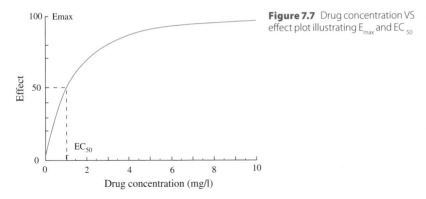

Figure 7.7 Drug concentration VS effect plot illustrating E_{max} and EC_{50}

effect will also vary. Using these terms together, we can say that agonists have both affinity for, and efficacy at, receptor sites but while antagonists have affinity for receptor sites, they do not directly exert an effect. As described above, drugs have to be present in certain concentrations in the body in order to exert their effects. The term *potency* is used to describe the relative concentration (or dose) of a drug that has to be present in order to produce the desired effect. The more potent a drug, the less that has to be administered for a given effect. These concepts can be shown in Figure 7.8 where the drug response (effect) is plotted against log concentration for drugs of varying agonist effect, efficacy and potency.

As described above, antagonists stop or block a system by occupying a receptor site. The body will still be producing its own natural chemical messengers (ligands) but these cannot exert their usual effect at a receptor site in the presence of the antagonist. Antagonists can be *competitive* or *non-competitive* in nature. A competitive antagonist will compete with the natural ligand for receptor sites and form a reversible bond. As more drug antagonist is made available (by, for example, giving further doses and increasing the concentration of drug in the body's circulation) the antagonist is able to occupy more receptors than the agonist and

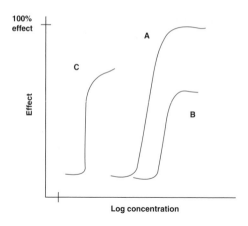

Figure 7.8 Agonists, efficacy and potency. Drug A is a full agonist as it exerts maximal effect when all receptors are occupied, while drug B is only a partial agonist. Drugs A and B are equipotent but A is more efficacious. Drug C is more potent than A or B

more of the body's own natural response is blocked. In order to overcome this effect, more of the body's own natural agonist needs to be made available in order to compete with the antagonist for these receptor sites, i.e. competition needs to be set up between agonist and antagonist. A non-competitive antagonist also forms a bond at a receptor site but often this bond is almost irreversible. Therefore, no matter how much of the natural agonist is present, the antagonist still exerts its effect.

Over time the processes of metabolism and excretion mean that the antagonist concentration declines naturally and the effect is lost, unless continuous dosing of the patient is maintained.

Drugs acting at enzyme systems

Some drugs have their effect by altering the effect of the body's enzyme systems. Sometimes, the drug may resemble the enzyme's natural substrate and so competition is set up between the drug and the natural substrate for binding to the enzyme. Other times, the drug may bind irreversibly to the enzyme's active site, therefore rendering it unable to carry out its usual function. An example of a drug acting on an enzyme system is that of the angiotensin converting enzyme inhibitors (ACEIs), which block the enzymatic conversion by renin of the physiologically inactive angiotensin I to the vasoconstrictor angiotensin II. These ACEIs are used to control blood pressure by preventing vasoconstriction as well as having other indications.

Drugs acting at ion channels

Sometimes in the body a system is controlled by cells allowing the selective movement of certain ions across cell membranes, e.g. calcium or potassium ions, which sets up an electrical potential gradient across the membrane. Anything that alters this selective movement across a cell membrane can alter this electrical potential and therefore affect that body system. For example, calcium channel blocker drugs (e.g. nifedipine and diltiazem) act by blocking natural channels across cell membranes, which under certain situations allow the passage of calcium ions across smooth muscle cells. This results in an altered electrical potential and therefore an altered physiological response, in this case a reduced force of contraction of smooth muscle in the heart and ultimately a reduction in hypertension.

Drugs acting on carrier mechanisms

In the first section of this chapter we discussed the process of active transport systems that allowed certain ions and molecules to be maintained at different concentrations in different cells of the body. These active transport systems are energy-dependent carrier mechanisms and some drugs can interfere with these mechanisms. Examples include digoxin, which blocks the H^+/K^+ pump in the heart, and the proton pump inhibitor drugs, like omeprazole, which block the Na^+/K^+ pump in the gastric mucosa.

Further in-depth discussions of the concepts described in this section can be found in the further reading at the end of this chapter.

As we can see the concepts of pharmacokinetics and pharmacodynamics are very complex. It is important that prescribers have at least a basic understanding of these, in order to be able to predict and individualise drug therapy. They are also important in understanding how drugs interact and why drugs can exert unwanted or adverse effects.

Drug interactions and adverse drug reactions

Drug interactions

It is not difficult to understand just as the body's own systems do not work in isolation, but interact to maintain a homeostatic environment, that when two or more drugs are administered to a patient, there is the potential for these drugs to interact with each other. Although pharmacologically two or more drugs may interact, the interaction may not always lead to a clinically significant effect. Drug interactions that are clinically significant can be either harmful or sometimes beneficial and may not occur in every patient.

It is not possible for prescribers to be aware of every potential drug interaction. By understanding how drugs can interact, in whom these interactions are more likely to occur and which drugs are most likely to be involved, they can apply this knowledge to their prescribing practice. If in doubt, prescribers should always check the literature or seek specialist advice before prescribing multiple drugs for patients.

Who is at risk of drug interactions?

Any patient receiving two or more drugs is at potential risk of a drug interaction. However, the greater the number of drugs a patient receives, the greater the number of potential drug interactions. There are also some groups or individuals who may be more susceptible to drug interactions. These include:

The elderly

The elderly population generally receive a number of different drugs for the treatment of multiple conditions or to reduce the potential risk of future morbidities. Coupled with this fact, they may also have declining physiological functions, for example, renal function may be impaired to some degree. For these reasons *polypharmacy* (the prescribing of a number of different drugs to one individual) increases the potential for drug interactions in this group of patients.

Seriously ill patients

Patients who are seriously ill or who have undergone a serious intervention, e.g. organ transplant, may be receiving numerous drugs and may have altered physiological functions as a result of their illness or condition.

Patients who receive prescriptions from more than one prescriber

In the modern NHS a number of professions are now able to train to prescribe either as independent prescibers (IPs) or as supplementary prescribers (SPs). These professions include nurses, pharmacists and some allied health professionals (e.g. physiotherapists). Therefore a patient may consult a number of different clinical practitioners and receive a prescription. Unless there is good communication between all prescribers and clear records are maintained, there is the potential for drug interactions to occur, due to lack of information being available at the time of prescribing.

Other groups

Other patient groups who are at potential risk include those taking drugs with a narrow therapeutic index, those with renal or hepatic impairment, patients taking over-the-counter medication which is not documented in their records and those who require long-term drug therapies for a specific disease or condition.

Which drugs are more likely to be involved in drug interactions?

While theoretically any two drugs could interact, not all do and even if they do, the outcome may not be clinically significant. There are some drugs which for a number of reasons are more likely to be involved in a drug interaction. These include drugs with a narrow therapeutic index, those that act on the cytochrome P450 enzyme system, drugs that require the same protein carrier type and drugs that act on the same receptor type. A list of drug interactions is given in the *British National Formulary* (BNF 2009) and a prescriber must decide which may be clinically significant in their specific patient.

How do drugs interact?

There are many ways in which drugs can interact with one another. In this section, we will only consider drug interactions that occur in the body and not those which can occur before the drug is administered to a patient, due to, for example, storage conditions. In describing how drugs can interact, we will refer to concepts and processes described earlier in this chapter.

Pharmacokinetic drug interactions

Drug interactions may occur at any stage of ADME. Regardless of at which stage the interaction takes place, the overall effect is to alter the concentration of drug in the plasma and therefore either increase or decrease its effect.

Absorption

Anything that interferes with the absorption of a drug from its site of administration will alter the bioavailability of the drug, and ultimately, its effect. The most common type of drug interaction due to alteration of absorption occurs in the gastrointestinal tract. Some drugs may bind to others, if given at the same time and so prevent the absorption of one of the drugs, e.g. antacids may reduce the absorption of some commonly used antibiotics, hence the warnings that are put onto medicine bottles to avoid taking antacids at the same time as certain antibiotics. Some drugs may slow gastric emptying and so prolong the time it takes for another drug, given at the same time, to exert its effect. In other situations, giving a drug that increases gastric motility, e.g. metoclopramide, may adversely affect the absorption of a drug that requires gastric acid to break down its outer layer in order to activate the drug. For example, some enteric-coated drugs require a certain length of exposure to the acid environment of the stomach, in order to release the active drug. Earlier in this chapter, the concept of enterohepatic circulation was discussed in relation to the oral contraceptives, and the interaction between this reabsorption process and antibiotics was also described.

Distribution

Earlier in this chapter, the factors that effect drug distribution were described and it was noted that only free drug is pharmacologically active. Drugs bound to plasma proteins are inactive. Some drugs are very heavily protein-bound and if they are given at the same time as another highly protein-bound drug, competition will exist between the two drugs for the same protein binding sites. This may mean that the concentration of either drug as free drug may be increased or decreased, depending on which drug binds to the most protein binding sites. This may have no clinically significant effect but in certain situations the effect could be very significant. An example of this type was discussed above under the heading of protein binding where the interaction of warfarin and tolbutamide was described in relation to concentrations of circulation plasma proteins.

Metabolism

Earlier in this chapter, the CYP450 enzyme system was briefly described. The fact that certain drugs could induce or inhibit this system was discussed, with examples. If a patient is stabilised on a drug, for example phenytoin, and then an enzyme-inhibiting drug is given to that patient, e.g. erythromycin, then the metabolism of the phenytoin may be reduced (due to erythromycin inhibiting the enzymes needed to metabolise phenytoin, leading to higher concentrations circulating in the body). As phenytoin is a drug with a narrow therapeutic index, small changes in its plasma concentrations can cause toxicity, as in this example, or lead to a reduction in its effect. Prescribers should always consult the *British National Formulary* (BNF 2009) for clinically important enzyme inducers or inhibitors and their potential drug interactions.

Excretion

Some drugs can alter the excretion of other drugs. For example, NSAIDs like ibuprofen or diclofenac can reduce the renal excretion of lithium. Again, lithium is a drug with a narrow therapeutic index, so reducing its excretion can have serious toxic effects.

Pharmacodynamic drug interactions

These can sometimes be predicted by knowing the mechanism of action of the drugs involved. There are too many to describe in this chapter but some common examples are described below.

Asthmatic patients are advised to avoid ß-blocker drugs. This is because ß-receptors are present in the bronchioles and in the heart. So, in this example, an asthmatic patient relies on the agonist effect of salbutamol on $ß_2$-receptors in the bronchioles to keep their airways open. If a ß-blocker is given to this patient, there is the potential that it may block not only $ß_1$-receptors in the heart, but also some $ß_2$-receptors in the bronchioles. If this happens, it will antagonise the effect of the salbutamol and the patient may experience wheezing, or worse, the effect may precipitate an asthma attack due to reduced effect of the salbutamol. Although drugs are formulated to be more *selective* for one type of receptor than another, e.g. $ß_1$-selective ß-blockers are formulated so that they act on the $ß_1$-receptors in the heart but not those $ß_2$-receptors in the bronchioles and smooth muscle. However, there is always the possibility that selectivity is not 100% – i.e. *selectivity* is relative.

ACEIs and NSAIDs can interact due to the effect that both increase fluid and K^+ concentrations. Digoxin used in controlling atrial fibrillation is affected by K^+ concentrations, so potassium-sparing diuretics, e.g. amiloride, can interact with digoxin.

Prescribers should always consult the *British National Formulary* (BNF 2009) for clinically important drug–drug interactions before prescribing for any patient taking more than one drug.

Adverse drug reactions (ADRs)

Any drug given to a patient can cause an unintended harmful effect. This effect can be described as an *adverse drug reaction* (ADR). ADRs are very common and are thought to occur in 10–20% of all patients prescribed drugs. ADRs are thought to be implicated in approximately 4% of all hospital admissions and are the cause of up to 10% of all GP consultations. One UK-based study over a nine-week period concluded that of the 840 screened admissions to an adult acute ward, 85 (10.1%) were drug-related and 52% of these were caused by an ADR (Bhalla et al. 2003). Another UK-based study analysed over 18 000 hospital admissions over six months and found that 1,225 admissions were related to an ADR (Pirmohamed et al. 2004).

The problem with ADRs is that they may not be recognised as such but instead considered to be an integral part of the patients' disease progression. As with drug interactions, it is not possible for a prescriber to have knowledge of all possible ADRs (particularly as some are idiosyncratic in nature). Prescribers should be vigilant and consider ADRs as one of the possible options when patients experience problems.

What are adverse drug reactions?

The classification of ADRs can be very complex and can be explored in more depth in the further reading suggested at the end of this chapter.

ADRs can be classified into two types, *Type A* and *Type B*.

Type A reactions

These are often predictable from the drug's pharmacology and are caused by an excessive or inadequate response to a drug. These can be the result of pharmacokinetic or pharmacodynamic problems. This type of ADR is often predictable, dose-related and can be managed, often by simple dose alteration. In fact, many commonly documented side effects of drugs are Type A adverse drug reactions, an unwanted but predictable response to a drug. Some examples of Type A reactions include aminoglycoside (e.g. gentamicin) hearing impairment due to drug accumulation in patients with poor or impaired renal function and NSAID-related peptic ulcer, due to the blockade of prostaglandin synthesis, which protects the stomach lining.

Type B reactions

These are idiosyncratic in nature, not predictable from the drug's pharmacology and therefore unrelated to the dose of the drug. Although they are not as common as Type A reactions, they are clinically very important, as the effect of a Type B ADR can be very serious. An example would be an anaphylactic reaction to a therapeutic dose of penicillin.

Who is at risk of adverse drug reactions?

As discussed above, some ADRs are completely idiosyncratic and cannot be predicted. However, prescribers should be extra cautious in certain patient groups, including the elderly and the very young (due to altered pharmacokinetic and pharmacodynamic processes), patients with renal or liver impairment or disease and patients with a known genetic predisposition, e.g. glucose 6-phosphate dehydrogenase, who can suffer haemolysis when given certain drugs.

Reporting adverse drug reactions

Many rare Type B ADRs will not show up in pre-marketing drug testing, as not enough patients are exposed to the drug. As some ADRs are so rare, a drug may need to be given to 10 000 or even 100 000 patients to pick up one adverse incident, or some drugs may need to be chronically administered for a long period in order for an ADR to manifest. This is why reporting of ADRs is very important. All prescribers have a responsibility to report a potential ADR to the proper authorities. In the UK, the Medicines and Healthcare products Regulatory Agency (MHRA) collects data and reports of ADRs.

The Yellow Card scheme is run by the MHRA and the Commission on Human Medicines (CHM), and is used to collect information from both health professionals and the general public on suspected side effects or ADRs to a medicine. It is a voluntary reporting system and its continued success depends on the willingness of people to report suspected ADRs.

The MHRA accepts Yellow Card reports from anyone from the UK on both licensed and unlicensed medicines including:

- Prescription medicines.
- Over-the-counter (OTC) medicines.
- Herbal remedies.
- Cosmetic treatments.

Reporting an ADR to the MHRA can be done online or by using the yellow reporting cards which can be found at the back of the *British National Formulary* (BNF 2009). The MHRA collate information on ADRs from Yellow Card reporting and other sources and may decide to publish warnings and advice for prescribers regarding certain types of ADRs and how to minimise these. The MHRA may also take the decision to revoke a licence and withdraw a drug from the market, if it is felt to be in the public's best interests.

Individualising drug therapy

In the previous sections of this chapter, we have considered the basic principles and concepts with which prescribers should be familiar with in order to prescribe safely and effectively. A lot of the issues covered will be considered almost subconsciously by prescribers, e.g. in what form to administer a drug to a patient, but other issues may need more considered thought, e.g. are any of these drugs likely to interact?

What is important is that for every patient prescribed for, the prescriber should take an individual approach. No two patients will be alike and prescribers need to remember this. A diagrammatic representation of individualising drug therapy and the many issues that prescribers need to consider is shown in Figure 7.9.

Patients handle drugs differently once they have been administered and even when a drug reaches its site of action its effect may not be what was predicted. Patients may have co-morbidities which will impact on the expected drug effect, they may be taking other drugs which will interact, or they may experience an ADR which may or may not be predictable. It is hoped that by reading this chapter and the suggested further reading, new prescribers will have a better understanding of some of these basic principles and consider them appropriately in their practice.

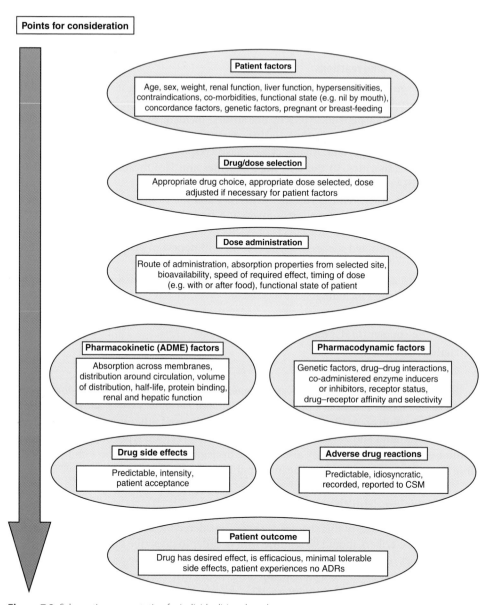

Points for consideration

Patient factors
Age, sex, weight, renal function, liver function, hypersensitivities, contraindications, co-morbidities, functional state (e.g. nil by mouth), concordance factors, genetic factors, pregnant or breast-feeding

Drug/dose selection
Appropriate drug choice, appropriate dose selected, dose adjusted if necessary for patient factors

Dose administration
Route of administration, absorption properties from selected site, bioavailability, speed of required effect, timing of dose (e.g. with or after food), functional state of patient

Pharmacokinetic (ADME) factors
Absorption across membranes, distribution around circulation, volume of distribution, half-life, protein binding, renal and hepatic function

Pharmacodynamic factors
Genetic factors, drug–drug interactions, co-administered enzyme inducers or inhibitors, receptor status, drug–receptor affinity and selectivity

Drug side effects
Predictable, intensity, patient acceptance

Adverse drug reactions
Predictable, idiosyncratic, recorded, reported to CSM

Patient outcome
Drug has desired effect, is efficacious, minimal tolerable side effects, patient experiences no ADRs

Figure 7.9 Schematic representation for individualising drug therapy

References

Bhalla, N., Duggan, C., Dhillon, S. (2003). The incidence and nature of drug-related admissions to hospital. *The Pharmaceutical Journal 270*: 583–586.

British National Formulary. (2009). London: BMJ Group and RPS Publishing.

Pirmohamed, M. et al. (2004). Adverse drug reactions as cause of admission to hospital: prospective analysis of 18 820 patients. *British Medical Journal 329*: 15–19.

Weatherall, D.J., Ledingham, J.G., Warrell, D.A. (eds). (2006). *Oxford Textbook of Medicine* (fourth edition). Oxford: Oxford University Press.

Further reading

Baxter, K. et al. (2008). Drug interactions and fruit juices. *The Pharmaceutical Journal* 281: 333.

Hawksworth, G.M. (2003). Drug metabolism. *Medicine 31*(8): 16–17.

McKinnon, J. (2004). A painless introduction to pharmacology for nurses. Part 1. *Nurse Prescribing 2*(1): 16–19.

McKinnon, J. (2004). A painless introduction to pharmacology. Part 2: therapeutics and metabolism. *Nurse Prescribing 2*(3): 122–126.

McLeod, H.L. (2003). Pharmacokinetics for the prescriber. *Medicine 31*(8): 11–15.

Monitoring skills

Part a – Asthma

Trisha Weller

Asthma is common in the UK, with over 5.2 million people with asthma, and more than 3 million receiving current treatment (National Asthma Campaign (NAC) 2001). Approximately 2.6 million people with asthma still have serious symptoms, mostly due to a failure of asthma management (Asthma UK 2004). The prevalence of asthma has risen over the last 30 or more years (British Thoracic Society (BTS) 2001) and the majority of asthma patients are cared for within primary care.

Asthma – the disease

Asthma is a reversible airways disease characterised by bronchoconstriction, inflammation, oedema and mucus production; more recent descriptions also include airways hyper-responsiveness. Asthma is reversible either spontaneously or with anti-asthma treatment.

The estimated prevalence rate of asthma in young children varies from 12.5% to 15.5%, while in adults current symptomatic asthma is reported by 7.8% of people (NAC 2001). There is a wide spectrum of disease severity, and treatment requirements vary. Control of asthma is assessed against a standard of (BTS/Scottish Intercollegiate Guidelines Network (SIGN) 2008):

- No daytime symptoms.
- No night-time awakening due to asthma.
- No need for rescue medication.
- No exacerbations.
- No limitation on activity including exercise.
- Normal lung function (in practical terms, forced expiratory volume in one second (FEV1) and/or peak expiratory flow (PEF) more than 80% predicted or best).

Nurse involvement in asthma management

Primary care-based nurses have been involved with asthma management since the General Medical Services contract (Department of Health and Social Security (DHSS) 1990) and the Health of the Nation White Paper (Department of Health (DoH) 1992). The General Medical Services contract (DoH 2003) for primary care rewards general practices financially if they provide a quality health service. This includes payment for the provision of asthma services as long as certain quality indicators are achieved. One of the quality indicators within the asthma domain requires a review of asthma patients within the last 15 months. Similarly, within an organisational domain of medicines management, patients who are prescribed more than four repeat medications should have a documented review of their medications in the preceding 15 months.

The British Guideline on the Management of Asthma (BTS/SIGN 2008) provides a framework for asthma treatment based on published research evidence; this guideline has helped to standardise asthma care in the UK. Asthma should be treated according to recommended guidelines and treatment reviewed as part of a structured review. This includes a review of symptoms with treatment stepped up as necessary and stepped down when control is good (BTS/SIGN 2008). The framework is divided into treatment steps for different age groups based on supporting evidence. These age groups are:

- Adults.
- 5–12 years.
- Under 5 years.

Supporting evidence for treatment is less clear under the age of 2 years and expert opinion should be sought where the diagnosis is in doubt.

New episodes of asthma are reported to be declining (Fleming et al. 2000) and it has been suggested that nurses have contributed to this decline (Weller et al. 2001).

It is essential that health professionals providing asthma care have had appropriate asthma training. The British Guideline on the Management of Asthma (BTS/SIGN 2008) states that 'in primary care, people with asthma should be reviewed regularly by a nurse or doctor with appropriate training in asthma management'. Asthma UK (previously NAC), in its Asthma Charter 2003, supports the right of patients to have access to a doctor or nurse who has had specific asthma training (www.asthma.org.uk).

Education for Health (www.educationforhealth.org.uk), formerly the National Respiratory Training Centre, is the leading respiratory education provider for primary care nurses in the UK and more than 11 000 nurses have successfully completed their accredited diploma level asthma module. As a result, this asthma module is frequently a stated requirement for practice nurses and many have considerable knowledge and clinical skills in asthma management.

Asthma treatment prior to independent and supplementary prescribing

Prior to independent and supplementary prescribing, many nurses involved in asthma management were already making treatment decisions but prescribing was still the responsibility of the general practitioner. In some situations, asthma-trained nurses may have had a more up-to-date knowledge of asthma than their medical colleagues!

Nurses involved in asthma chronic disease management were initially frustrated by early prescribing restrictions, which meant that they could prescribe for their asthma patients if they had eczema and/or rhinitis, but could not prescribe their asthma treatment (Medicines Control Agency (MCA) 2002).

Supplementary prescribing and asthma

Patients with asthma can now be assessed, reviewed and have their asthma medications prescribed by a nurse prescriber (NP). If using supplementary prescribing, the initial diagnosis needs to be confirmed by an independent prescriber (IP) who is a doctor. A clinical management plan (CMP) must be agreed by the IP and SP before supplementary prescribing begins: the patient must also agree and have an active role in this decision-making process. The British Guideline on the Management of Asthma provides evidence that an individual written asthma action plan (or self-management plan) detailing asthma treatment improves asthma outcomes (BTS/SIGN 2008). There is also evidence that an asthma-trained nurse can make a difference to clinical asthma outcomes (BTS/SIGN 2008; Dickinson et al. 1997).

Pharmacists and asthma monitoring

Community pharmacists have an important role monitoring asthma patients too, because they are often initially consulted for symptoms such as coughs and colds, and for 'over-the-counter' treatments. Colds can make asthma worse and a greater awareness of asthma monitoring and clinical management can enhance patient care.

The new contractual pharmacy contract has been introduced throughout the UK (http://www.dh.gov.uk/en/Publicationsandstatistics/Publications/PublicationsPolicyAndGuidance/DH_4109256; http://wales.gov.uk/news/archivepress/healthpress/2007/1421243/?lang=en; http://www.scotland.gov.uk/Publications/2004/06/19514/39165;http://www.dhsspsni.gov.uk/index/pas/non-medical-prescribing.htm).

Service provision is divided into essential, advanced and enhanced services. Advanced services include a medicine use review service, while the enhanced service include disease-specific medicines management services. Pharmacists must fulfil the correct criteria in order to provide more than the essential service. A sound clinical asthma management knowledge is an area that needs addressing, in order to maintain optimum care for asthma patients.

Pharmacists in England, Wales, Scotland and Northern Ireland are eligible to become independent and supplementary prescribers.

Asthma medications

There are three main groups of asthma medications. They are:

- Bronchodilators.
- Glucocorticosteroids.
- Leukotriene receptor antagonists (LTRAs).

A newer and different asthma medication is an anti IgE monoclonal antibody but it is not widely used.

Bronchodilators

These are divided into:

- Short-acting bronchodilators (beta$_2$ agonists), e.g. salbutamol and terbutaline.
- Anti-cholinergic medications, e.g. ipratropium bromide.
- Long-acting bronchodilators (long-acting beta$_2$ agonists), e.g. salmeterol and formoterol.
- Methylxanthines, e.g. theophyllines and aminophylline.

Short-acting bronchodilators: these are used for symptomatic relief on an as-required basis for wheeze, cough, breathlessness, chest tightness and if required prior to exercise. They are used in high doses in worsening and acute asthma. Common side effects are tachycardia and tremor and are usually dose related.

Anti-cholinergic medication: ipratropium bromide is used for the treatment of acute severe asthma where there has been an initial poor response to short-acting bronchodilators. It is nebulised with short-acting bronchodilators (BTS/SIGN 2008). Side effects include a dry mouth.

Long-acting bronchodilators: these are used as first line additional therapy to short-acting bronchodilators and low-dose corticosteroids. They should not be used to treat an acute asthma attack. Side effects are similar to short-acting bronchodilators.

There has been concern over the safety of long-acting beta agonists in the management of asthma following a report in 2005 by the Food and Drug Administration (FDA) in the United States (http://www.fda.gov/consumer/updates/asthmameds051308.html). This stated that there might be an increase in severe asthma episodes and asthma deaths with the use of long-acting beta agonists, however, they were used without inhaled corticosteroids, whereas in the UK they are not. A review of the evidence-based asthma guidelines by the Medicines and Healthcare products Regulatory Agency (MHRA) concluded long-acting beta agonists are safe to use, but only if they are used in addition to an inhaled steroid as per the asthma guidelines (BTS/SIGN 2008).

Methylxanthines: these are used as additional therapy when there is no response to the long-acting bronchodilator therapy. There is wide variability in the half-life of the drug. It is increased in heart failure, cirrhosis, viral infections and the elderly, and by drugs such as cimetidine, ciprofloxacin, erythromycin and oral contraceptives. It is decreased in smokers and chronic alcoholism and by drugs such as phenytoin, carbamazepine, rifampicin and barbiturates. There is a narrow therapeutic safety window for methylxanthines and regular blood monitoring should be instigated because of the potential for side effects, such as tachycardia, gastrointestinal disturbance, headache, insomnia and convulsions.

Glucocorticosteroids

There are five inhaled glucocorticosteroids available in the UK:

- Beclometasone.
- Budesonide.
- Fluticasone.
- Mometasone.
- Ciclesonide.

Inhaled steroids are the first line preventer therapy for asthma (BTS/SIGN 2008). The lowest dose possible should be used to control asthma symptoms. Local side effects of dysphonia and candidiasis occur rarely but are usually dose related. Systemic side effects are very rare in lower dose ranges (up to 800 micrograms beclomethasone dipropionate (BDP) or equivalent). Inhaled steroids need to be taken regularly to obtain maximum benefit.

Initially inhaled steroids are taken twice a day, except ciclesonide which is a once-a-day inhaled steroid. In mild asthma, the other inhaled steroids are slightly more effective if taken twice a day, but they can be considered on a once-daily basis once control has been established; however, this should be at the same total daily dose as the previous twice-a-day regimen (BTS/SIGN 2008).

It is important to remember that fluticasone is used at half the dose of beclometasone or budesonide. Several reports indicate the likelihood of more serious side effects of adrenal insufficiency at doses above 500 micrograms fluticasone per day (Todd et al. 1996; 2002). Current BTS/SIGN guidelines suggest an upper limit of 800 micrograms beclometasone or equivalent in children (BTS/SIGN 2008).

Hawkins et al. (2003) report that inhaled steroids can be reduced effectively in patients with moderate to severe asthma without compromising asthma control. This study supports current guideline recommendations that lower doses of inhaled steroids should be used. Health professionals monitoring asthma patients need to ensure that asthma review includes reducing asthma treatment to the minimum needed to control symptoms.

Steroid cards are not issued routinely to asthma patients on inhaled corticosteroids but those taking regular oral steroids must be issued with one. Supplies of these cards are available from the DoH.

Leukotriene receptor antagonists

LTRAs are oral therapies that are generally used in addition to inhaled steroids and following a trial of long-acting bronchodilators. In children from ages six months to five years, they can be used as first line preventer therapy. There are two products available in the UK – montelukast and zafirlukast. Montelukast is used more widely and is taken once daily at night. Side effects include gastrointestinal disturbance, dry mouth and very occasionally sleep disturbance. Montelukast has a role in the treatment of rhinitis where there is co-existing asthma but only in adolescents and adults.

Combination inhalers

Although there is no difference in efficacy when inhaled steroids and long-acting beta$_2$ agonists are used either separately or together, combination inhalers are useful. Once asthma control is stable there are a number of advantages. It:

- Ensures the separate drug components are always taken together.
- May improve adherence because only one inhaler is needed.
- Simplifies the medication regimen.

Additionally in adults at Step 3 of the BTS/SIGN asthma guidelines, whose asthma is not controlled using their regular combination inhaler treatment, the combination inhaler Symbicort can be used as a rescue inhaler. It is important patients are counselled when using this regimen.

Anti IgE monoclonal antibody

Omalizumab is the only available drug of this type and is given as a sub-cutaneous injection every 2–4 weeks. It binds with circulating immunoglobulin E (IgE), reducing levels of free serum IgE and is helpful for a specific group of individuals where allergy is an important cause of their asthma. Omalizumab is only initiated in specialist centres with experience of caring for severe and difficult asthma and there are strict prescribing criteria. Licensing restrictions limit its use to individuals from 12 years of age. Very careful monitoring is required, but in secondary care.

Asthma medications and pregnancy

Asthma patients who are pregnant should be treated the same way as those who are not pregnant. Asthma medications should be continued in pregnancy including the use of oral steroids if they are required. LTRAs are not indicated in pregnancy unless prior treatment has demonstrated them to be clinically effective (BTS/SIGN, 2008). It is important to monitor pregnant women with asthma more closely so any changes in asthma control can be addressed.

Table 8.1 Licensing age range for inhaled steroids

Drug	Age range
Beclometasone (Asmabec)	From 6 years
Beclometasone (Clenil)	Under 15 years always with a large volume spacer
Beclometasone (Pulvinal)	6 years and over
Beclometasone (Qvar)	12 years and over
Budesonide (Novolizer inhaler)	6 years and over
Budesonide (Pulmicort inhaler)	2 years and over
Budesonide (Turbohaler)	5 years and over
Ciclesonide	12 years and over
Fluticasone (Evohaler)	4 years and over
Fluticasone (Accuhaler) 250 mcg, 500 mcg	Not indicated for children
Fluticasone (Diskhaler) 250 mcg, 500 mcg	Not indicated for children
Fluticasone (Evohaler) 125 mcg, 250 mcg	Not indicated for children
Mometasone	From 12 years

Source: British National Formulary 58, September 2009
http://emc.medicines.org.uk/default.aspx accessed 27/1/2010

N.B. Qvar and Clenil are not interchangeable with CFC containing beclometasone inhalers and should be prescribed by brand name

Table 8.2 Licensing age range for long acting bronchodilators

Drug	Age range
Salmeterol	From 4 years
Formoterol (Oxis Turbohaler)	From 6 years
Formoterol (Atimos Modulite)	From 12 years
Formoterol (Easyhaler)	From 5 years
Formoterol (Foradil)	From 6 years

Source: British National Formulary 58, September 2009
http://emc.medicines.org.uk/default.aspx accessed 27/1/2010

Asthma medications in young children

Several asthma medications are unlicensed for the younger paediatric asthma patient because of the ages defined within the product licence. The Royal College of Paediatricians and Child Health (RCPCH) has published a policy statement on the use of unlicensed medicines, or licensed medicines for unlicensed applications, in paediatric practice (RCPCH 2003). The use of these medicines can be justified where they are the most appropriate medication, but parents of these children must be informed as to why this choice was made.

There are several drug strengths available for many of the different asthma medications, as well as a range of drug delivery systems. The higher drug strengths are not indicated for children over 12 years, but this raises the question as to 'what age defines a child?'. Licensing applications need to be more specific to avoid potential confusion for prescribers. Tables 8.1 and 8.2 illustrate the variable licensing age ranges of inhaled steroids and long-acting bronchodilators.

Table 8.3 Variable drug doses and relevant licensing age for combination asthma therapies

Seretide (Fluticasone + salmeterol)	Age range
Accuhaler device (100 mcg Fluticasone)	Over 4 years
Accuhaler device (250 mcg Fluticasone)	Over 12 years
Accuhaler device (500 mcg Fluticasone)	Over 12 years
Evohaler metered dose inhaler (50 mcg Fluticasone)	Over 4 years
Evohaler metered dose inhaler (125 mcg Fluticasone)	Over 12 years
Evohaler metered dose inhaler (250 mcg Fluticasone)	Over 12 years
Symbicort (Budesonide + formoterol)	**Age range**
Turbohaler (100/6 mcg)	Over 6 years
Turbohaler (200/6 mcg)	Over 12 years
Turbohaler (400/12 mcg)	Over 12 years
Fostair (Beclometasone + formoterol)	**Age range**
	Over 18 years

Source: British National Formulary 58, September 2009
http://emc.medicines.org.uk/default.aspx- accessed 27/1/2010

Table 8.3 illustrates the variable licensing ages for combination therapy of inhaled steroids and long-acting bronchodilators. This variability can lead to confusion for prescribers where the separate components have different licensing age ranges.

There is considerable variability in licensing age ranges for asthma medications. When new products first appear on the market, licensing indications are usually restricted to 12 years and over. This age range relates to the research studies carried out to obtain a product license. It does not mean that the products are unsafe below the stated age range; merely that there were no supporting studies when the product was first licensed.

Nurses monitoring asthma patients need to be aware not only of the medication required, according to current guidelines, but also product license indications. The MHRA advise that both Qvar and Clenil are prescribed by brand name, because of the different bioavailability of other beclometasone inhaler devices.

Monitoring adverse effects

Nurses can report drug side effects using the established Yellow Card system (Committee on Safety of Medicine (CSM/MCA 2002). This drug reporting system provides an early warning system to the Medicines and Healthcare products Regulatory Agency (MHRA) (previously known as the MCA and the CSM). The Yellow Card reporting system began in 1964 after the drug thalidomide was withdrawn, but reporting was limited to doctors, dentists, coroners and pharmacists, as well as the pharmaceutical industry. Inclusion of nurses within the current reporting system acknowledges the important monitoring role that nurses have in drug usage, especially within chronic disease management. Electronic submission is also possible, which facilitates easier and quicker submission of reports.

Newly licensed medications are monitored carefully by the MHRA and the CSM when they are first introduced or if there is a change in drug route or delivery system. These medications are indicated by a black triangle symbol in the *British National Formulary* (BNF) and the *Monthly Index of Medical Specialities* (MIMS). No upper time limit is set for this black triangle identification but these medications are usually reviewed after a minimum of two years.

Asthma monitoring

At each asthma review it is important to:

- Review any medication changes including dose alterations.
- Always ask the patient or carer what they are taking. This can be different to what has been prescribed.
- Be alert to possible medication side effects.
- Assess inhaler technique and modify technique when appropriate.
- Change inhaler device if the technique cannot be corrected.
- Consider the addition of a spacer device if high doses of inhaled steroid are used.
- Ensure plastic spacers are washed as per the BTS/SIGN 2008 recommendations.
- Ensure treatment follows national asthma guideline recommendations.
- Provide a written action plan tailored to the individual (BTS/SIGN 2008) and agreed with the independent medical prescriber and asthma patient.
- Issue a peak flow meter and determine appropriate peak flow values with the patient as part of the asthma action plan, for those with:
  - Brittle or life-threatening asthma.
  - Previous admissions to hospital.
  - Unscheduled care for asthma emergencies.
  - Frequent courses of oral steroids.
  - Treatment at Step 3 of the asthma guidelines (BTS/SIGN, 2008) and above.
- Provide a follow-up review date.

Summary

Independent and supplementary prescribing enhances the care that asthma patients receive. Monitoring of respiratory symptoms and drug therapy is essential and should be carried out by a health professional with established expertise in asthma management. National asthma guidelines should be followed and a multidisciplinary approach to care is essential.

Further information

- Asthma training. Further information is available from Education for Health (formerly National Respiratory Training Centre). www.educationforhealth.org.uk. Tel: 01926 493313.
- Asthma UK (previously National Asthma Campaign). www.asthma.org.uk.
- British Guideline on the Management of Asthma. http://www.brit-thoracic.org.uk/ClinicalInformation/Asthma/AsthmaGuidelines/tabid/83/Default.aspx
- Steroid cards are available from: DoH, PO Box 777, London SE1 6XH.

References

Asthma UK (2004). Living on a knife edge. http://www.asthma.org.uk/all_about_asthma/publications/living_on_a_knife_ed.html

British Thoracic Society (2001). *The Burden of Lung Disease. A Statistics Report from the British Thoracic Society*. London: BTS.

British Thoracic Society/SIGN (2008). British Guideline on the Management of Asthma. Revised ed. *Thorax* 63(Suppl IV).

Committee on Safety of Medicine/MCA (2002). *Extension of the Yellow Card Scheme to Nurse Reporters*. London: CSM/MCA.

Department of Health (1992). *The Health of the Nation: A Strategy for Health in England*, London: HMSO.

Department of Health (2003). *Investing in General Practice: The New General Medical Services Contract*. London: DoH.

Department of Health and Social Services (1990). *General Practice in the National Health Service. A New Contract*. London: HMSO.

Dickinson, J., Hutton, S., Atkin, A. et al. (1997). Reducing asthma morbidity in the community: the effect of a targeted nurse-run asthma clinic in an English general practice. *Respiratory Medicine* 91: 634–640.

Fleming, D.M., Sunderland, R., Cross, K.W. et al. (2000). Declining incidence of episodes of asthma: a study of trends in new episodes presenting to general practitioners in the period 1989–1998. *Thorax* 55(8): 657–661.

Hawkins, G., McMahon, A.D., Twaddle, S. et al. (2003). Stepping down inhaled corticosteroids in asthma: a randomised controlled trial. *British Medical Journal 326*: 1115–1118.

Medicines Control Agency (2002). *Proposals for Supplementary Prescribing by Nurses and Pharmacists and Proposed Amendments to the Prescription Only Medicines (Human Use) Order 1997*. MLX 284. London: MCA.

National Asthma Campaign (2001). Out in the open. *Asthma Journal 6*(3) (suppl): 1–14.

Royal College of Paediatricians and Child Health (2003). The use of unlicensed medicines or licensed medicines for unlicensed applications in paediatric practice. In: *Medicines for Children* (second edition). London: RCPCH Publications Limited, pp. xvi–xviii.

Todd, G., Dunlop, K., McNaboe, J. et al. (1996). Growth and adrenal suppression in asthmatic children treated with high-dose fluticasone propionate. *Lancet 348*: 27–29.

Todd, G.R.G., Acerini, C.L., Buck, J.J. et al. (2002). Acute adrenal crisis in asthmatics treated with high-dose fluticasone propionate. *European Respiratory Journal 19*: 1207–1209.

Weller, T., Booker, R., Walker, S. (2001). Declining incidence of episodes of asthma: letter. *Thorax 56*(3): 246.

Part b – Coronary heart disease

Paul Warburton

Coronary heart disease (CHD) is the leading cause of mortality in the developed world. In the UK, diseases of the heart and circulatory system are the main cause of death, accounting for almost 198 000 deaths in 2006 (Allender et al. 2008). CHD is the most common cause of death in the UK, killing over 94 000 people in 2006 and almost 31 000 of these occurred before the age of 75 (BHF 2008). The death rate from CHD in the UK has been falling steadily since the 1970s, however, despite these improvements it remains amongst the highest in the world.

CHD is a common condition that has a significant impact on both individuals with the condition and society in general. For individuals it is frequently fatal and often debilitating, leading to a reduction in quality of life. For society the economic cost is enormous; CHD is estimated to cost the UK economy £9 billion annually (Allender et al. 2008), yet it is largely preventable. The underlying pathology of CHD is usually atherosclerosis and this develops over many years, often without any signs or symptoms.

Table 8.4 Risk factors for coronary heart disease

Fixed	Modifiable
Age	Smoking
Male sex	Hypertension
Family history	Raised cholesterol
	Diabetes
	Obesity
	Poor diet
	Sedentary lifestyle

There are a number of well recognised and understood risk factors for CHD; these are the same as those for other cardiovascular disease (CVD), therefore risk calculators now reflect this. The modification of these risk factors has been conclusively shown to reduce mortality and morbidity in both individuals with or without a previous history of cardiovascular disease. Risk factors can be categorised as fixed or modifiable (see Table 8.4). The fixed risk factors of age, male sex or a family history of CHD cannot be corrected.

When discussing the risk of developing a condition such as CVD, it is important to distinguish between relative risk (the proportional increase in risk) and absolute risk (the actual chance of an event). The risk of developing CVD multiplies when there is more than one risk factor present. Therefore people with a combination of risk factors have a greater risk of developing CVD. For example, a man aged 40 who smokes 30 cigarettes per day and has an elevated serum cholesterol level of 8 mmol/litre is far more likely to die in the next ten years from CVD than a non-smoking woman of the same age with a low serum cholesterol level. However, the likelihood of this happening is still low. He therefore has a high relative risk of developing CVD but a low absolute risk.

Fixed risk factors

The risk of an individual developing CVD rises with age and males are affected in larger numbers than females (Allender et al. 2008). Family history is an important fixed risk factor; the Framingham study (Schildkraut et al. 1989) has shown that a history of death due to CVD in parents of an individual was associated with a 30% increased risk of developing CVD. Indeed, all CVD risk calculators now reflect in their equations the increased risk of developing CVD in those individuals with a first-degree relative with premature CVD (men < 55 years and women < 65 years). This increased risk may be due to genetic factors or the effects of a shared environment (such as a similar diet) and habits (such as smoking). As CVD often runs in families, the first-degree relatives of patients with premature CVD and those with family members who have hyperlipidaemia should be risk assessed for developing CVD. This should be done using a recognised risk calculator, such as the Joint British Societies Cardiovascular Risk Charts (JBS 2005), and intervention provided where necessary following the appropriate evidence.

Modifiable risk factors

Smoking

Smoking is the single most avoidable cause of chronic diseases including CVD in the UK. Tobacco smoke is also responsible for the death of more people in the UK than any other avoidable cause

(RCP 2005). There is a strong, consistent and dose-related relationship between cigarette smoking and CVD. Smoking promotes the build up of coronary plaques and can lead to premature plaque rupture and subsequent myocardial infarction. It is estimated that about 'half of all regular smokers will eventually be killed by their habit' (Doll et al. 2004) and that 20% of CVD deaths in the UK are attributable to smoking. Despite the well-recognised relationship between smoking and CHD, in Great Britain in 2006, 23% of men and 21% of women smoked (BHF 2008).

Hypertension

In Western societies, the average systolic and diastolic blood pressure rises with age. In England in 2006, 31% of men and 28% of women had hypertension or were being treated for the condition (BHF 2008). This showed some overall improvement from previously recorded figures. Hypertension is defined as a systolic blood pressure of 140 mmHg or over or a diastolic blood pressure of 90 mmHg or over (JBS 2005). The risk of developing CHD and other vascular disorders is related directly to both systolic and diastolic blood pressure levels; this risk rises continuously across the pressure ranges. Therefore, a reduction in blood pressure leads to a decreased risk of not only CHD but also other circulatory conditions, such as stroke and renal dysfunction.

Hypertension is diagnosed following the measurement of blood pressure on three separate occasions. In more than 95% of cases of hypertension, no underlying cause is found. This is known as essential, or primary, hypertension. In 70% of those with essential hypertension, another family member is affected.

Patients with isolated systolic hypertension (systolic pressure ≥ 160 mmHg with diastolic pressure ≤ 90 mmHg), especially those aged over 60, are at an increased risk of developing CVD including stroke and coronary events. Such patients should have their CVD risk assessed and be treated in the same way as other patients with hypertension.

In the majority of cases, the discovery of hypertension will mean a lifetime of monitoring and treatment with antihypertensive medications. However, general lifestyle measurements can prove successful in the reduction of blood pressure and all such patients should be asked about the lifestyle factors that may influence their blood pressure. Appropriate verbal, written and audio-visual guidance should then be offered to address issues, such as excessive alcohol and salt consumption, improving diet, correcting obesity and increasing exercise levels. Regular exercise improves physical conditioning and can also lead to a lower blood pressure.

Diet and obesity

Consumption of a healthy diet is associated with a reduced risk of developing cardiovascular and other diseases. In general, dietary recommendations include a reduction in fat intake, particularly saturated fats, reduction in salt intake and an increase in the intake of carbohydrates and fruit and vegetables (DoH 1994). It is with this in mind that the DoH introduced the 'five a day' recommendation of five portions of fruit and vegetables daily. It is estimated that adopting such a diet can help to reduce the risk of developing chronic diseases such as CVD by up to 20% (WHO 2003).

The number of people who are overweight or obese in the UK continues to rise and has roughly doubled since the mid-1980s; this is probably due to the increasing calorific intake and increased sedentary lifestyles within the population. Within the general population of England in 2006, 67% of men and 57% of women were overweight or obese (BMI of 25 kg/m^2 or more) (Joint Health Surveys Unit 2008). Being overweight or obese is an important risk factor in the development of hypertension, diabetes and chronic diseases including CHD. The incidence of type 2 diabetes due to insulin resistance is associated with obesity and is a strong risk factor for the development of CHD (Yusuf et al. 2004).

Diabetes

Diabetes is a common disorder that is known to affect approximately 2.5 million people in the UK with around 90% of these having type 2 diabetes (Diabetes UK 2008). This figure does not include those that have undiagnosed diabetes; this is estimated to be 3.1% of men and 1.5% of women aged over 35 in England (DoH 2004). Diabetes is an important independent risk factor for developing vascular complications and CVD. Patients with type 2 diabetes have a significantly increased risk of having a cardiovascular event and the associated mortality is up to five times greater in people with diabetes that those without it (WeMeReC 2005). The benefits of rigorous blood pressure (Blood Pressure Lowering Treatment Trialists' Collaboration 2005) and blood sugar control (UK Prospective Diabetes Study Group 1998) in diabetics has now been conclusively demonstrated. The assessment and treatment of modifiable risk factors in diabetics and the associated primary prevention of CVD is therefore essential. This patient group benefits from being treated as if they have existing CVD and risk calculators now reflect this fact.

Hypercholesterolaemia

Although there is clear evidence that an individual's risk of developing CVD is directly related to their total blood cholesterol levels, low density lipoprotein (LDL) cholesterol is a more accurate predictor of cardiovascular events. Statin therapy reduces the relative risk of major events by 20% for every 1 mmol/L reduction in LDL cholesterol (Baigent et al. 2005). The high density lipoprotein (HDL) level is inversely related to cardiovascular risk, therefore as the HDL increases, the risk of developing CVD is reduced. Lowering LDL cholesterol and raising HDL cholesterol slows progression of the process of atherosclerosis and reduces the risk of developing CVD. Lowering the concentration of both total cholesterol and LDL cholesterol is effective in the primary and secondary prevention of CVD. Cholesterol levels can be reduced by changes in diet, increased physical activity and cholesterol-lowering drugs. For the *primary* prevention of CVD in people without type 2 diabetes, no target levels for total or LDL cholesterol levels are currently recommended (NICE 2008).

Target levels for total cholesterol for the *secondary* prevention of CVD in individuals with established CVD have been revised downwards in the UK since the publication of the National Service Framework for CHD (DoH 2000). The new ideal targets are to lower cholesterol by 30% or to reach 4 mmol/L for total cholesterol and 2 mmol/L for LDL cholesterol, whichever is the greater (JBS 2005; NICE 2008).

Risk calculators

There are a number of well-recognised cardiovascular risk calculator tools available to estimate the absolute risk of developing CVD, most of which have evolved from tools designed to estimate risk of developing CHD alone. These tools are primary prevention aids designed to be used for individuals who have not already developed CHD or other major atherosclerotic disease. The most widely used CVD risk predictor chart in the UK is the Joint British Societies Cardiovascular Risk Prediction Chart (JBS 2005).

Risk calculators provide an indication of an individual's 10-year risk of developing CVD and this is expressed as a percentage figure. Lower risk individuals are those with a < 10% risk of developing CVD and higher risk individuals are defined as those with a 10-year risk of developing CVD ≥ 20%.

Risk calculators are a useful aid to clinical decision making when considering pharmacological intervention, such as lipid-lowering or antihypertensive therapy, however, they should not replace clinical judgement. They are also valuable in illustrating to patients the benefits of risk factor modification, such as stopping smoking, controlling blood pressure or reducing cholesterol levels.

Medications used in primary prevention of coronary heart disease

As with all prescribing, when prescribing medications to reduce the risk of developing CVD, the principles of prescribing (NPC 1999) should be used. It is important to involve the patient in the decision-making process and discuss with them the treatment options available to address their individual risk factors. The purpose, benefits, effects and possible side effects of the medication(s) should be explained along with how and when it should be taken. The alternatives to the prescribed treatment should also be discussed.

Antihypertensives

The purpose of treating hypertension is to effectively lower blood pressure to within recognised acceptable limits, reduce the risk of complications and improve survival. Antihypertensives should reduce blood pressure and be well tolerated. There are a wide range of evidence-based medications available to treat hypertension and selection is usually based upon individual patient factors, however, combination therapy of more than one medication is often required to attain adequate blood pressure control. These are usually added in a step-wise manner until control is achieved. Angiotensin-converting enzyme inhibitors (ACE-Is), calcium-channel blockers (CCBs) or low-dose thiazide diuretics are considered to be initial treatment choices, although β-blockers may be indicated where CHD is also present.

ACE inhibitors

Angiotensin-converting enzyme inhibitors (ACE-Is) are very effective antihypertensives and are recommended as an effective first line choice in hypertensive patients who are under 55 years of age and not black (i.e. of African or Caribbean ethnicity). ACE-Is control blood pressure by inhibiting the conversion of angiotensin 1 to angiotensin 2, they are well tolerated and have a good side effect profile. The most common side effect is a dry persistent cough. ACE-Is should be used with care in patients with impaired renal function. Renal function and electrolytes should be monitored in all patients before commencing an ACE-I and again 7–10 days after starting or increasing the dose.

Angiotensin-II receptor antagonists

Angiotensin-II receptor antagonists (AIIAs) or angiotensin-II receptor blockers (ARBs) have an action similar to that of ACE-Is but do not cause the persistent dry cough associated with ACE-Is. Currently there is no compelling evidence to suggest benefit of using an AIIA instead of an ACE-I and they are therefore usually used in those patients unable to tolerate an ACE-I due to a persistent cough. As with ACE-Is, AIIAs should be used with care in patients with impaired renal function. Renal function and electrolytes should be monitored in all patients before commencing an AIIA and again 7–10 days after starting or increasing the dose.

Beta blockers

β-blockers have been shown to be less effective than other antihypertensive agents in reducing blood pressure. They are also associated with an increased risk of developing diabetes, especially if used with a thiazide diuretic. Therefore the use of β-blockers as a first line agent to control blood pressure is no longer recommended (NICE 2006) although they may be suitable for younger people in certain circumstances, for example, if ACE-Is are contraindicated (e.g. in pregnant women) or are not tolerated.

Calcium channel blockers

Calcium channel blockers (CCBs) are effective antihypertensives and interfere with the inward displacement of calcium ions through the cell membranes. They are recommended as a first choice of therapy for hypertensive patients who are black or aged 55 years or over (NICE 2006). Different CCBs work different sites of action and therefore there are important differences in the actions and effects of various CCBs. They are usually well tolerated although common side effects include ankle swelling, flushing and headache.

Thiazide diuretics

Low-dose thiazide diuretics inhibit sodium reabsorption in the distal convoluted tubule and are effective and cost-effective antihypertensives. There is good evidence supporting their use and benefits and they are recommended as a first choice of therapy for hypertensive patients who are black or aged 55 years or over (NICE 2006).

Antiplatelet medications

Antiplatelet medications reduce platelet aggregation in the arterial circulation and may inhibit thrombus formation. There is strong evidence that the use of aspirin in people who do not have established vascular disease reduces the risk of developing CVD including myocardial infarction (Antithrombotic Trialists' Collaboration 2002). In asymptomatic high-risk individuals aged 50 years or over, low-dose aspirin is beneficial in the primary prevention of CVD when the 10-year risk is $\geq 20\%$. In patients who experience a true hypersensitivity reaction with aspirin, clopidogrel may be used as an alternative antiplatelet drug (CKS 2008) although it is considerably more expensive.

Cholesterol-lowering medications

There are a number of medications available to reduce cholesterol levels. These include statins, fibrates, bile acid sequestrants and anion-exchange resins. Statins are the first choice and the mainstay of cholesterol-lowering treatment in both the primary and secondary prevention of CVD as there is conclusive evidence of their ability to reduce both primary and secondary cardiovascular events. There are a number of effective statins available with varying degrees of potency, however, initial treatment for primary and secondary prevention of CVD should be with simvastatin 40 mg once daily (NICE 2008). Statins competitively inhibit an enzyme involved in the synthesis of cholesterol called 3-hydroxy-3-methylglutaryl coenzyme A (HMG CoA) reductase. In those patients who are unable to tolerate a statin, a fibrate or anion-exchange resin may be considered to reduce cholesterol. The combined use of a statin with another cholesterol-lowering medication, such as a fibrate, anion-exchange resin or nicotinic acid, is not recommended due to the increased risk of side effects.

Smoking cessation

Smoking cessation interventions can reduce ill health and prolong life and are cost effective. Nicotine replacement therapy (NRT) and bupropion are effective aids to smoking cessation in individuals who are motivated to stop and who smoke more than ten cigarettes each day. NRT is the pharmacological intervention of choice in smoking cessation and it is available in different formulations including skin patches, chewing gum, nasal spray and tablets. It can improve the success rate of quitting by 50–70% (Stead et al. 2008). The success of such therapies is increased when supported by a clinic, such as an NHS Stop Smoking Service (NICE 2006).

Recommendations for primary prevention

Individuals without diagnosed CVD who have a risk of ≥ 20% of developing CVD over 10 years should be identified and structured care provided to reduce this risk. Current UK guidance (JBS 2005; NICE 2008; SIGN 2007) recommends that all people aged 40 or above, or at any age in those individuals with a first-degree relative with premature CVD or hypercholesterolaemia, should have their risk of developing CVD assessed. Calculation of risk should then be reassessed at least every five years (JBS 2005). This strategy allows the identification of those at increased risk of developing CVD and the implementation of appropriate evidence-based intervention.

In such individuals the following steps should be taken:

- Smokers should be advised to give up and supported with appropriate intervention, such as nicotine replacement therapy.
- A healthy lifestyle should be promoted. Assessment of individual risk factors should be made and information given as appropriate regarding modifiable risk factors, such as diet, physical activity, weight and alcohol consumption. The information provided and its format should be personalised to individual needs.
- Where blood pressure exceeds 140/80 mmHg, advice and treatment to maintain blood pressure below this level should be given.
- A statin should be added if the person's estimated CVD risk is 20% or more.

The identification of an individual as being at increased risk of developing CVD leads to many challenges for that individual and the prescriber. Patterns of behaviour, such as smoking, a sedentary lifestyle and diet are usually lifelong and often require professional assistance in achieving change. Referral to services, such as a smoking cessation service or dietician, may prove useful in achieving change. Education and support should be provided for all patients along with explanation of the rationale, benefits and effects of their therapy as, despite being asymptomatic, they may be required to continue with lifelong medications. Concordance with medications can therefore be a problem, particularly when polypharmacy is needed or if side effects occur. The management of patients at high risk of developing CVD requires a collaborative approach to change and the benefits of these changes should be explained and reiterated to each patient.

References

Allender, S., Peto, V., Scarborough, P. et al. (2008). *Coronary Heart Disease Statistics.* London: British Heart Foundation.

Allender, S., Scarborough, P., Peto, V. et al. (2008). *European Cardiovascular Disease Statistics.* Brussels: European Heart Networks.

Antithrombotic Trialists' Collaboration (2002). Collaborative meta-analysis of randomised trials of antiplatelet therapy for the prevention of death, myocardial infarction and stroke in high-risk patients. *British Medical Journal 324*(7329): 71–86.

Baigent, C., Keech, A., Kearney, P.M. et al. Cholesterol Treatment Trialists' (CTT) Collaborators (2005). Efficacy and safety of cholesterol-lowering treatment: prospective meta-analysis of data from 90 056 participants in 14 randomised trials of statins. *Lancet, 366*: 1267–1278.

Blood Pressure Lowering Treatment Trialists' Collaboration (2005). Effects of different blood pressure-lowering regimens on major cardiovascular events in individuals with and without diabetes mellitus: results of prospectively designed overviews of randomized trials. *Archives of Internal Medicine 165*(12): 1410–1419.

Clinical Knowledge Summaries (2008). Antiplatelet treatment, http://www.cks.nhs. uk/antiplatelet_treatment (accessed 31 December 2008).

Department of Health (1994). *Nutritional Aspects of Cardiovascular Disease. Report of the Cardiovascular Review Group of the Committee on Medical Aspects of Food Policy.* London: HMSO.

Department of Health (2000). *National Service Framework for Coronary Heart Disease.* London: Department of Health.

Department of Health (2004). *Health Survey for England 2003.* London: The Stationery Office.

Diabetes UK (2008). Diabetes prevalence 2008, http://www.diabetes.org.uk/Professionals/Inf ormation_resources/Reports/Diabetes-prevalence-2008/ (accessed 31 December 2008)

Doll, R., Peto, R., Boreham, J. et al. (2004). Mortality in relation to smoking: 50 years' observations on male British doctors. *British Medical Journal, 328*: 1519–1527.

Joint British Societies (2005). JBS 2: Joint British Societies' guidelines on prevention of cardiovascular disease in clinical practice. *Heart, 91*(Suppl 5): v1–v52

Joint Health Surveys Unit (2008). *Health survey for England 2006. Cardiovascular disease and risk factors.* Leeds: the Information Centre, http://www.ic.nhs.uk/webfiles/publications/ HSE06/HSE%2006%20report%20VOL%201 %20v2.pdf (accessed 30 December 2008).

National Institute for Health and Clinical Excellence (2006). Public health intervention guidance no.1. Brief interventions and referral for smoking cessation in primary care and other settings. March 2006, http://www. nice.org.uk/nicemedia/pdf/SMOKING-ALS2_FINAL.pdf (accessed 1 January 2009).

National Institute for Health and Clinical Excellence (2008). Lipid modification. Cardiovascular risk assessment: the modification of blood lipids for the primary and secondary prevention of cardiovascular disease. Clinical Guideline 67. May 2008, http:// www.nice.org.uk/nicemedia/pdf/CG067NIC EGuideline.pdf (accessed 1 January 2009).

National Prescribing Centre (1999). Signposts for prescribing nurses – general principles of good prescribing. Liverpool: National Prescribing Centre, http://www.npc.co.uk/nurse_ bulletins/sign1.1.htm (accessed 31 December 2008).

Royal College of Physicians Tobacco Advisory Group (2005). Going smoke-free. The medical case for clean air in the home, at work an in public places, http://www.rcplondon.ac.uk (accessed 31 December 2008).

Schildkraut, J.M., Myers, R.H., Carrison, R.J. (1989). Coronary risk associated with age and sex or parental heart disease in the Framingham Heart Study. *American Journal of Epidemiology, 64*: 555–559.

Scottish Intercollegiate Guidelines Network (2007). Risk estimation and the prevention of cardiovascular disease, http://www.sign.ac.uk /pdf/sign97.pdf (accessed 30 December 2008).

Stead, L.F., Perera, R., Bullen, C. et al. (2008). Nicotine replacement therapy for smoking cessation (Cochrane Review). *The Cochrane Library.*John Wiley & Sons, Ltd, http:// www.thecochranelibrary.com (accessed 1 January 2009).

UK Prospective Diabetes Study Group (1998). Effect of intensive blood-glucose control with metformin on complications in overweight patients with type 2 diabetes (UKPDS 34). *Lancet 352*(9131): 854–865

WeMeReC (2005). Type 2 diabetes important aspects of care. WeMeReC, http://www.wemerec.org/Documents/ Bulletins/ Diabetes_bulletin.pdf (accessed 30 December 2008).

World Health Organization (2003) *Diet, Nutrition and the Prevention of Chronic Diseases.* Geneva, WHO, http://whqlibdoc.who.int/trs/who_TRS_916.pdf (accessed 30 December 2008).

Yusuf, S., Hawken, S., Ôunpuu, S. et al. on behalf of the INTERHEART Study Investigators (2004). Effect of potentially modifiable risk factors associated with myocardial infarction in 52 countries (the INTERHEART study): case-control study. *Lancet, 64*: 937–952.

Part c – Diabetes

Jill Hill

Diabetes is becoming very common worldwide. In the UK, it was estimated in 1989 that there were 1.3 million people living with the condition. This figure was predicted to rise to 3.1 million by 2010 (Amos et al. 1997). The increasing prevalence is primarily caused by a rise in the number of people developing type 2 diabetes, and is closely related to the increasing proportion of the population that is overweight or obese. The diabetes epidemic has serious implications for the use of NHS resources as diabetes is costly, estimated in 2001 as consuming about 5–10% of the total NHS budget (DoH 2001). About 40% of this cost is consumed in the management of preventable complications of diabetes (Baxter et al. 2000). All patients with diabetes, whether type 1 or type 2, are at risk of developing diabetic complications. These include microvascular (retinopathy, neuropathy and nephropathy) and macrovascular complications (myocardial infarction, angina, stroke and peripheral vascular disease). Successful management of blood glucose, blood pressure, lipids and other risk factors reduces the risk of diabetes complications (Stratton et al. 2000).

Diabetes is defined as a condition characterised by a chronically raised plasma glucose concentration (hyperglycaemia), due to a complete or relative lack of insulin to maintain blood glucose within normal levels (Watkins 1998). Despite this very clear definition, diagnosing diabetes may not be simple. Being diagnosed with diabetes has major implications for that person's way of life, so it is essential that there is no doubt about the diagnosis. The World Health Organization has provided clear criteria for establishing the presence of diabetes and impaired glucose intolerance (WHO 1999).

The diagnosis of type 1 diabetes is usually clear cut. A short history of osmotic symptoms (thirst and polyuria) with significant weight loss, with a venous sample in the diagnostic range, will confirm the diagnosis. The presence of ketones in the urine or blood confirms that the patient has type 1 rather than type 2 diabetes. Approximately 15% of people with diabetes have type 1, with most presenting before the age of 30 (but not always). It is caused by an autoimmune-mediated destruction of the insulin-producing beta cells in the pancreas gland, eventually causing a complete lack of insulin. Treatment is always, therefore, insulin replacement therapy.

Type 2 diabetes is a complex condition that is usually a manifestation of the metabolic syndrome. This includes hypertension, dyslipidaemia, central obesity, clotting abnormalities and inadequately compensated insulin resistance. Patients usually require medication to address most or all of these factors and are prescribed a large number of tablets. Unfortunately, there is evidence that many patients do not take these tablets as prescribed (Donnan et al. 2002). Type 2 diabetes is progressive. In the early stages (indeed for years before diagnosis), tissue sensitivity to insulin action decreases (insulin resistance) and there is a compensatory increase in insulin production by the beta cells. Beta cell failure is a later feature in the natural history of the condition. The typical treatment history of type 2 diabetes, progressing from diet and lifestyle modification alone, then oral hypoglycaemic agents, to eventual insulin therapy, reflects this progression from insulin resistance to beta cell failure (Wright et al. 2002).

Gestational diabetes is a condition of glucose intolerance which presents during pregnancy, due to inadequate beta cell compensation for the insulin resistance resulting from pregnancy hormones. This may require insulin therapy but the condition disappears at the end of pregnancy. However, women who develop gestational diabetes are at significant increased risk of developing type 2 diabetes later in life.

MODY (Mature Onset Diabetes in the Young) is a complex collection of diabetes inherited as an autosomal dominant gene. Patients are usually young, and some types may have a low risk of complications. MODY is relatively rare.

An NSF (National Service Framework) for diabetes was launched in 2001, setting 12 standards of care that should be achieved by 2013 (DoH 2001). These standards cover all aspects of diabetes care, from prevention, early identification and routine care, to specialist areas, such as management of diabetes in children and pregnancy. There are also a number of technology appraisals and guidelines issued by NICE that support good diabetes practice.

Non-insulin treatments for blood glucose

Whether their diabetes is managed with tablets or insulin or no medication, people with diabetes need to adopt a healthy eating plan (Diabetes UK 2003), increase daily physical activity and avoid damaging lifestyle behaviours, to achieve control of blood glucose, cholesterol, blood pressure and weight. Some patients with type 2 diabetes may manage to maintain normal glycaemia with lifestyle alone, at least initially. Typically, however, patients with type 2 diabetes require oral hypoglycaemic agents to initially improve insulin sensitivity and stimulate beta cell production of insulin, but eventually insulin therapy to supplement their endogenous insulin. Guidelines for the management of type 2 diabetes have recently been revised by the National Institute of Health and Clinical Excellence (NICE 2008).

Metformin is the only available example of the biguanides. It is usually the first agent of choice unless it is contraindicated (significant renal impairment or severe heart or liver failure can cause lactic acidosis) or the patient is very symptomatic. Gastrointestinal side effects are common, but slow-release metformin may improve tolerance. It is particularly useful in overweight patients with type 2 diabetes, as it does not stimulate beta cell production of insulin and is therefore unlikely to cause weight gain or hypoglycaemia.

Sulphonylureas stimulate insulin release from the beta cells in the pancreas. The main side effects are weight gain and hypoglycaemia. People who have erratic meal patterns may benefit from taking a **prandial regulator** instead of a sulphonylurea as these agents, taken just before a meal, stimulate the beta cells for a shorter period of time to control post-prandial glucose levels.

The **thiazolidinediones**, pioglitazone and rosiglitazone, improve insulin sensitivity by reducing peripheral insulin resistance. They are contraindicated in patients who have a past history of heart failure as these agents can cause fluid retention which can exacerbate underlying heart failure. There has been concern about rosiglitazone following a meta-analysis showing an increased risk of myocardial infarction in patients using this agent (Nissan and Wolski 2007). There is no evidence to show this is the case with pioglitazone: indeed the PROactive study showed some benefit for patients who had already had a myocardial infarction (Dormandy et al. 2005).

There have been two recent additions to the choice of non-insulin therapy for people with type 2 diabetes: the **gliptins** and **GLP-1 mimetics**. At the time of writing, there are two GLP-1 mimetics available: exenatide (Byetta), which is a twice-daily injection; and liraglutide (Victoza), which is a daily injection. Incretin hormones are produced in the small intestine and have various effects including suppressing post-prandial glucagon production and causing a feeling of satiety (and therefore suppressing appetite). Use of a GLP-1 mimetic is recommended for patients with type 2 diabetes, who have a BMI of 35 or greater (30 or greater if hypoglycaemia must be avoided, or a co-existing co-morbidity-like sleep apnoea makes further weight gain very undesirable) and who would otherwise need insulin or a glitazone. There was some concern initially about an increased risk of pancreatitis in patients using exenatide, so patients starting a GLP-1 mimetic should be warned about symptoms of acute abdominal pain. The gliptins are DPP-IV inhibitors and there are three available at the time of writing: sitagliptin (Januvia); vildagliptin (Galvus); and saxagliptin (Onglyza). DPP-IV is an enzyme that deactivates natural incretin hormone. Gliptins' mode of action, therefore, is to prolong the action of endogenous incretin hormones.

Insulin therapy

Patients with type 1 diabetes, and eventually most people with type 2 diabetes, require insulin therapy. There are four companies supplying a variety of insulin in the UK, which can be grouped by onset and duration of action. Most insulins are available in disposable pens or cartridges to fit durable pens, with some also available in vials for use with a syringe. A limited supply of pork and beef insulins is still available.

Rapid-acting analogue insulin (Apidra, Novorapid and Humalog) mimics the short 'bursts' of insulin produced after a carbohydrate load in someone without diabetes. They are injected just before a meal (or can be given at the end of a meal), start to work within 15 minutes and last for up to 3–5 hours. Patients with type 1 diabetes are usually encouraged to adjust the amount of these mealtime insulins with the amount of carbohydrate they have eaten. A week-long course called DAFNE or Dose Adjustment For Normal Eating (DAFNE 2002) has been recommended by NICE for patients with type 1 diabetes (NICE 2003).

Short-acting insulin (e.g. Humulin S, Hypurin Porcine Neutral). These are injected 20 minutes before meals but have a longer duration than the rapid-acting analogues, lasting up to 8 hours.

Intermediate insulin is cloudy and needs to be resuspended at least ten times before use. It is used once or twice daily with mealtime insulin to give a basal bolus regime or may be used with oral agents in people with type 2 diabetes. Insulatard, Insuman Basal and Hypurin Porcine Isophane are examples.

There are two **basal analogue** insulins: Detemir and Glargine. These can provide a long-acting background insulin (up to 24 hours with one injection). Unlike the traditional background insulins, these insulins are clear like the mealtime insulins so patients need to check they are giving the correct insulin if they are using both, as they look similar. They can be used with oral agents in type 2 diabetes or as part of a multiple-dose injection (or basal bolus regime) in patients with type 1 diabetes.

Table 8.5 Targets recommended by NICE for most people with type 2 diabetes (NICE 2009)

Parameter	Target
Glycosylated haemoglobin (HbA1c)	6.5–7.5% (the lower target for newly diagnosed type 2 diabetes)
Blood pressure	<140/80 (<130/80 if microvascular complications present)
Total cholesterol	<4 mmol/L
LDL cholesterol	<2 mmol/L

There are a limited range of **insulin mixtures** available: Mixtard 30; Humulin M3; Hypurin Porcine 30/70 mix; and Novomix 30 (in which 30% of the insulin is either short- or rapid-acting insulin), and Humalog Mix 25 and Humalog Mix 50 (in which 25% or 50% respectively is rapid-acting insulin). These insulins are usually given twice a day, before breakfast and the evening meal, but can also be used three times a day.

Patients using insulin should be advised on correct injection technique (into subcutaneous fat usually on the abdomen, thighs and buttocks), safe disposal of needles and the recognition of hypoglycaemia symptoms and how to treat these appropriately. Rapid-acting carbohydrate (like dextrose tablets or Lucozade) should be readily available at all times. Glucagon 1 mg injections may be helpful for use by carers of patients with no awareness of hypoglycaemia who have severe hypoglycaemic episodes.

The Diabetes Control and Complications Trial (DCCT 2003) was a key trial demonstrating that intensive glucose management reduces the risk of microvascular complications in people with type 1 diabetes. The UK Prospective Diabetes Study (UKPDS 1998) demonstrated a similar result in people with type 2 diabetes. However, management of lipids and blood pressure is also very important, particularly in the prevention of macrovascular complications in patients with type 2 diabetes.

Diabetes monitoring

All people with diabetes should be offered annual retinopathy screening and a diabetes annual review (DoH 2001). These identify early signs of diabetes complications at a stage when treatment may slow progression (e.g. laser treatment to prevent blindness), identify risk factors that lead to complications (e.g. abnormal cholesterol levels or blood pressure), and are an opportunity for patient education and feedback. Diabetic medication is also reviewed, doses titrated, new medications added and treatments that are not tolerated or have become contraindicated (e.g. Metformin if creatinine raises above 150 mmol/L) are removed. The annual review is usually performed by the patient's GP and/or practice nurse. Diabetes features significantly in the points that can be achieved in the Quality and Outcomes Framework of the General Medical Services contract (Kenny 2005). The review should include at least the following:

- Blood tests for lipid profile, glycaemic control and renal function (creatinine and estimated glomerular filtration rate).
- Blood pressure.
- Weight and body mass index.
- Nerve sensitivity (using a 10 g monofilament), circulation (pedal pulse palpation) and general examination of the feet.

Recommended targets for most people with type 2 diabetes are given in Table 8.5.

References

Amos, A.F., McCarty, D.J., Zimmet, P. (1997). The rising global burden of diabetes and its complications: estimates and projections to the year 2010. Diabetic Medicine; *14*(Suppl 5): S1–S85.

Baxter, H., Bottomley, J., Burns. E. et al. (2000). CODE-2 UK. The annual direct costs of care for people with type 2 diabetes in Great Britain. *Diabetic Medicine*; *17*(Suppl 1): 13.

DAFNE Study Group (2002). Training in flexible, intensive insulin management to enable dietary freedom in people with type 1 diabetes: dose adjustment for normal eating (DAFNE) randomised controlled trial. *British Medical Journal 325*: 746–749.

Department of Health (2001). *National Service Framework for Diabetes*: Standards. London: Stationery Office.

Diabetes Control and Complications Trial (1993). Research Group. The effect of intensive treatment of diabetes on the development and progression of long-term complications in insulin-dependent diabetes mellitus. *New England Journal of Medicine 329*(14): 977–986.

Diabetes UK (2003). Nutrition Committee of the Diabetes Care Advisory Committee of Diabetes UK. The implementation of nutritional advice for people with diabetes. *Diabetic Medicine 20*: 786–807.

Donnan, P.T., MacDonald, T.M., Morris, A.D. (2002). Adherence to prescribed oral hypoglycaemic medication in a population of patients with type 2 diabetes: a retrospective cohort study. *Diabetic Medicine 19*: 279–284.

Dormandy, J.A., Charbonnel, B., Eckland, D.J.A. et al. (2005). Secondary prevention of macrovascular events in patients with type 2 diabetes in the PRO active Study (PROspective pioglitAzone Clinical Trial In macroVascular Events): a randomised controlled trial. *Lancet 366*: 1279–1289.

Kenny, C. (2005). Diabetes and the quality and outcome framework. *British Medical Journal 331*: 1097–1098.

National Institute for Health and Clinical Excellence (2003). *Guidance on the Use of Patient Education Models for Diabetes. Technical Appraisal 60*. London: NICE.

National Institute for Health and Clinical Excellence (2008). *Type 2 Diabetes: the Management of Type 2 Diabetes. NICE Clinical Guideline 66*. London: NICE.

National Institute for Health and Clinical Excellence (2009). *Type 2 Diabetes: the Management of Type 2 Diabetes. NICE Clinical Guideline 87*. London: NICE.

Nissan, S.E., Wolski, K. (2007). Effect of rosiglitazone on the risk of myocardial infarction and death from cardiovascular causes. *New England Journal of Medicine 356*: 2457–2471.

Stratton, I.M., Adler, A.I., Andrew, H. (2000). Association of glycaemia with macrovascular and microvascular complications of type 2 diabetes (UKPDS 35): prospective observational study. *British Medical Journal 321*: 405–412.

United Kingdom Prospective Diabetes Study 33 (1998). Intensive blood-glucose control with sulphonylureas or insulin compared with conventional treatment and risk of complications in patients with type 2 diabetes. *Lancet 352*: 837–853.

Watkins, P. (1998). *ABC of Diabetes*. London: BMJ Publishing Group.

World Health Organization (1999). *Definition, Diagnosis and Classification of Diabetes Mellitus and its Complications. Part 1. Diagnosis and Classification of Diabetes Mellitus*. Geneva: World Health Organization.

Wright, A., Burden, A.C., Paisley, R.B. et al. (2002). Sulfonyl inadequacy: efficacy of addition of insulin over 6 years in patients with type 2 diabetes in the UK Prospective Diabetes Study (UKPDS 57). *Diabetes Care 25*: 330–336.

Promoting concordance in prescribing interactions

Sue Latter

The introduction and expansion of non-medical prescribing is part of modernising the health service to make it accessible and responsive to patient needs. Increasing numbers of nurses, pharmacists and allied health professionals are now exercising their prescribing powers across a wide range of healthcare settings, and, since 2006, prescribing across the range of formulary medicines. This increases the points of access that patients have for obtaining medicines. However, gaining access to medicines from practitioners is unlikely to improve patients' health *per se*. Increasing access must be combined with a prescribing consultation in which the communication and interaction that occurs enables patients to take their medicines effectively to benefit their health.

Using the evidence base for effective prescribing, when effectiveness is measured in terms of potential health benefit, must include not only a consideration of the pharmacological evidence, but also the communication with patients that is required for effective medicine taking. The communication processes and attitudinal principles that are believed to embody an effective partnership model of prescribing are known as 'concordance'.

This chapter gives an overview of the evidence base for the concept of concordance and draws out the implications from research for the new generation of prescribers. It will begin by defining concordance and tracing its history and relationship to the concepts of 'compliance' and 'adherence'. A review of research into both compliance and concordance is followed by an outline of the reasons why practitioners who are independent (IPs) and/or supplementary prescribers (SPs) need to incorporate the principles of concordance into their practice. An overview of the skills and competencies that prescribing professionals need in order to adopt concordance in practice will then be presented. This is followed by a section on a review of research that has investigated nurses' and other healthcare professionals' concordance in practice.

What is concordance?

The term 'concordance' is used to refer to a partnership approach to interactions about medicines between healthcare professionals and patients. Philosophically and practically, it is used in place of the terms 'compliance' and 'adherence' as goals of medicine interactions, as the latter reflect an inappropriate emphasis on professional dominance and instructing or persuading the patient to comply or adhere to what the healthcare professional perceives to be important in medicine taking. Compliance and adherence also refer to the intended *outcomes* of medicine interactions, whereas concordance is about what happens in the *process* of an interaction, but with important links to effective outcomes of the interaction.

The term 'concordance' was first introduced in 1997 by the Royal Pharmaceutical Society of Great Britain (RPSGB), and has been defined as an approach to prescribing and taking medicines which is based on partnership:

> The patient and the healthcare professional participate as partners to reach an agreement on the illness and treatment. Their agreement draws on the experiences, beliefs and wishes of the patient to decide when, how and why to use medicines. Healthcare professionals treat one another as partners and recognise each other's skills to improve the patient's participation (Medicines Partnership 2003).

From this definition, it can be seen that there is a requirement to share experiences about medicines between the healthcare professional and the patient, and to reach an agreement and work in a co-operative way. Concordance is no different than adopting a partnership approach to other aspects of care and treatment that are provided for patients, but the term itself has come to be commonly used in relation to medicines management and prescribing interactions.

The promotion of concordance as the best practice approach within prescribing interactions has arisen for a number of reasons, including the fact that there remains a significant clinical and healthcare problem associated with medicine use, and the evidence base indicates that concordance is an effective way of helping to reduce this problem.

The prescribing problem

Patients do not always take medicines as prescribed and this phenomenon has been described as 'non-compliance'. Current estimates indicate that up to 50% of people living with long-term medical conditions do not take their medicines as prescribed (DoH 2000). Patients can be non-compliant in a number of different ways and it is important to be aware of these. Vermeire et al. (2001) highlight some of the stages and opportunities for non-compliance:

- Receiving a prescription, but not having it made up at pharmacy (primary non-compliance).
- Taking an incorrect dose.
- Taking the medication at the wrong times.
- Forgetting one or more doses of the medication.
- Stopping the treatment too soon, by ceasing to take the medication sooner than the prescriber recommended or failing to obtain a repeat prescription (secondary non-compliance).

Deliberately or unintentionally not taking medicines as prescribed may have impacts on both patients' health and that of their families or carers, and also impacts on the efficient and effective use of healthcare resources. The origins of this continuing problem are multi-factorial, as Marinker and Shaw (2003) point out: 'Patients do not comply with medication for several reasons. Non-compliance may be unintentional or involuntary. It may relate to the quality of information given, the impact of the regimen on daily life, the physical or mental incapacity of patients, or their social isolation.'

It is also important to realise that the impact of not taking medicines as intended by the prescriber may be perceived as either positive or negative by patients, and as such needs to be understood within the context of each individual's beliefs and lifestyle. The perceived impact of not taking medicines as prescribed may also differ between the patient and the healthcare professional prescriber. Furthermore, the perceived and actual impact of 'non-compliant' medicine taking may be more or less open to negotiation within a prescribing encounter. For example, a person may choose to take a lower dose of the medicine than has been prescribed because he or she wishes to manage the unpleasant side effects caused by the medication, and prefers to accommodate the attenuated and incompletely controlled symptoms of the illness than experience side effects. This example of non-compliance may be mediated within a prescribing encounter if the patient's views and beliefs on current management and medication are sought in an non-judgemental way, understood and perhaps an alternative medication offered with fewer side effects. Alternatively, another patient may cease to take their prescribed medication before completing the course because they generally hold negative and (scientifically) incorrect views about the medicine and they have become asymptomatic in regard to their illness. Again, the 'non-compliance' may be open to negotiation if the prescriber is able to elicit the patient's views about the action of the medicine and negotiate these, together with providing information about the significance of lack of symptoms.

This begins to suggest that 'non-compliance' is multidimensional, is best understood individually, may have negative impacts on both the patient's health and that of their family or carers as well as the efficient and effective use of healthcare resources, and that resolution of these issues demands a partnership approach to interactions in which the patient's views are sought in a non-judgemental manner and understood as a basis for possible negotiation.

Effective interventions – the evidence base

The evidence base for practice in this area is incomplete, but suggests that interventions required to address this issue are also multifactorial and complex, and that a concordance approach is likely to be one of the most effective strategies that a prescriber can adopt to influence and promote effective medicine taking. An overview of the evidence base for effective medicine interactions is given below.

Compliance research

From the 1970s to the 1990s, research into medicine taking was driven by the professional need to understand and predict non-compliance and to evaluate interventions that promoted compliance. The emphasis was on what needed to be done in order for patients to follow prescriptions as health professionals intended; characteristics of non-compliant patients were sought as well as the best methods of improving compliance. It is perhaps because the research questions driving this field of enquiry were too simplistic, and did not include research into patients' perspectives on the process and influences on medicine taking, that definitive answers to the question of compliance and how to ensure it were never found. That is to say, working from a professionally defined agenda (compliance), without taking account of patients' perspectives, is not likely to yield very conclusive results in understanding how to prescribe medicines effectively. Nevertheless, it is useful here to present a summary of what others have distilled from these decades of compliance research, before moving on to research focusing on concordance and its effectiveness.

Both Haynes et al.'s (2008) Cochrane review of interventions to promote adherence and Vermeire et al.'s (2005) Cochrane review of research into adherence in type 2 diabetes reach similar conclusions about both what is known in this area and the strength of the evidence base from which this knowledge derives. The authors concluded that no one single intervention has been shown to be effective in promoting adherence and that current interventions for adherence in long-term medical conditions are complex or multifactorial, and not very effective. Vermeire et al. (2005) found that nurse-led interventions, home aids, diabetes education, pharmacy-led interventions, adaptation of dosage and frequency of medication taking all showed a small effect on a variety of outcomes, including HbA1C, and therefore have some limited evidence to support their use in practice.

However, it is important to contextualise these strategies by reiterating Vermeire et al.'s (2001; 2005) more general observations from their reviews, that conclusions about what works are inconsistent across research studies, researchers have used a variety of outcome measures and adherence instruments and the research is often methodologically flawed. In their earlier review of adherence strategies across a range of clinical conditions, Vermeire et al. (2001) conclude that studies have led to partial and conflicting conclusions and that, to date, there is no evidence that any one method improves adherence better than another. They also comment on the lack of any theoretical framework to test interventions and notable gaps in the research base, such as that focusing on patient perspectives and the use of qualitative methods, to better understand what promotes adherence.

This review of compliance or adherence research highlights that the causes of and solutions to the issue of non-compliance are elusive and unlikely to be discovered through a lens that focuses only on a professionally determined perspective. What should the new generation of non-medical prescribers learn from these decades of research? Perhaps it is important to be aware of the repertoire of strategies, such as those outlined above, that have accrued *some* evidence to suggest that they may enhance 'compliance', even if this is incomplete and only partially understood. Nurses, pharmacists and allied health professionals, prescribing independently or in supplementary mode, may then draw on these strategies selectively and appropriately as part of an individualised approach to their prescribing interactions with patients.

The research review of Vermeire et al. (2001) also includes research and other literature on the effectiveness of characteristics of what is now known as concordance, and this evidence is reviewed below.

The evidence base for concordance

It is widely advocated that part of the repertoire of interventions necessary for effective medicine taking is a 'partnership approach' to the medicines consultation itself. But what evidence do we have for the effectiveness of this strategy, and how does it compare with the evidence for the other interventions that have been outlined above? In short, the evidence base for recommending a concordance approach to medicine interactions is also incomplete, but research in this area does suggest that concordance produces positive outcomes for patients. The reasons for recommending concordance as the preferred approach to interactions are also practical, ethical and philosophical, as will be outlined below.

Firstly, what is the research evidence that underpins concordance? Both research into theoretical models predictive of health behaviour and the impact of health professionals' communication skills are relevant here. The RPSGB's (1997) recommendations about concordance were underpinned by the importance of health beliefs in predicting medicine taking. They suggest that the most salient influences on medicine taking are patients' beliefs about medications and about medicines in general, and these therefore need to be elicited in the prescribing encounter as part of a concordance approach. This is supported by Horne et al.'s (2005) conclusions from their review of evidence into concordance and adherence, that 'the main development in this body of research over the last decade has been an increasing recognition of the importance of patients' "common sense" beliefs about their illness and treatment as the causes of non-adherence'. A recent synthesis of evidence derived from qualitative studies on medicine taking also supports this: patients' inaccurate beliefs about medicines were identified as the main reason why patients resist medicines and self-regulate their regime (Pound et al. 2005). Beliefs may include, for example, whether patients perceive a medicine as necessary for maintaining health, as well as concerns about possible adverse consequences, such as side effects, dependency or long-term harm. Shaw et al. (2005) point out that these beliefs are strongly influenced by the information that patients receive from health professionals.

There is then accumulating evidence to suggest that health beliefs about medicines and 'common sense' beliefs about illness, its causes and treatment can help us to explain medicine taking behaviour. Therefore, the necessity of exploring these within the prescribing interaction becomes clear – perhaps as a precursor to negotiation or the offer of information or explanation by the healthcare professional. This negotiation between the beliefs and priorities of, on the one hand, the patient, and on the other, the healthcare professional prescribing the medicine, is the essence of concordance. It is a respect for each party's knowledge and experiences that defines the concordance process.

The research evidence for the positive impact of concordance-orientated communication skills also points to the need to use this approach in practice. Cox et al. (2003) conclude from their review of communication between patients and healthcare professionals about medicine taking that concordance communication, such as encouraging patient participation and listening attentively to patients' views and concerns, may lead to improved outcomes, including enhanced adherence and satisfaction. Vermeire et al. (2001) also conclude that 'the literature contains sufficient evidence on the relationship between aspects of communication and the outcomes of patient satisfaction, recall and compliance for positive correlations to be made'. Similarly, Carter et al. (2003) conclude from their review, *A Question of Choice – Compliance in Medicine Taking*, that 'the available evidence, though incomplete, supports the view that holistic, patient-centred approaches – like concordance (patient–professional partnership in prescribing and medicines management) – are required to address poor compliance'.

The research evidence here does seem to point then to the importance of using communication skills to promote partnership and concordance in practice in pursuit of effective prescribing interactions.

The promotion of concordance is also a reflection of the philosophical shift within policy and practice generally towards greater user involvement and participation. The increasing interest in promoting partnership in healthcare professional–patient interactions is reflected in, for example, the Expert Patient Programme (DoH 2001), which highlights the need to make use of the expertise and experience of patients in managing their chronic diseases, such as asthma, arthritis and diabetes. This programme too is based not only on an ideology of partnership, but also on evidence which indicates that promoting self-efficacy and patient ability to take control over managing their own illness is more effective than healthcare professionals trying to do it for them. Information, choice and partnership are also key concepts in *High Quality Care for All: NHS Next Stage Review Final Report* (DoH 2008).

To summarise, the rise in popularity of concordance as an approach to medicine interactions reflects both the evidence base about effective interventions for medicines management and a philosophical stance, reflected in key contemporary policy, that places patient participation and partnership at the heart of healthcare, including medicines management.

What are the skills and knowledge required to practice concordance?

A closer examination of the published literature on the principal components of concordance begins to highlight what knowledge and skills IPs and SPs might require in order to put concordance into practice effectively.

The Medicines Partnership (2003) outlines three essential components of concordance:

1. *Patients have enough knowledge to participate as partners.* This involves offering patients information about medicines that is clear, accurate, accessible, sufficiently detailed and tailored to individual needs.
2. *Prescribing consultations involve patients as partners.* This means that patients are invited to talk openly about their priorities, preferences and concerns about medicine taking and treatment. Professionals explain the rationale for, and the characteristics of, the proposed treatment. Patients and health professionals jointly agree on a course of treatment that reconciles as far as possible the professional's recommendations and the patient's preferences. The patient's and the professional's understanding of what has been agreed is checked, as well as the patient's ability to follow the agreed treatment.
3. *Patients are supported in taking their medicines.* This requires that all opportunities be taken to discuss medicines issues and that healthcare professionals share medicines information effectively with one another. It also means that medications are reviewed regularly, with patients' participation, and that practical difficulties in taking medicines are addressed.

This suggests that skills in information giving and explanations about medicines, as well as using communication skills to elicit patient perspectives, are indicated.

The National Prescribing Centre's (NPC 2001) outline of prescribing competencies also reflects the importance of concordance as the preferred method of communication within prescribing consultations, and highlights skills and knowledge similar to those identified by Medicines Partnership (2003) above. More recently, the Medicines Partnership (2007) has developed a framework of shared decision-making competencies for achieving concordance in consultations: the framework outlines the skills and competencies that prescribers should use in order to enhance the quality and likely impact of their prescribing consultations on patient medicine taking. Table 9.1 outlines some examples of these.

Table 9.1 highlights that what is required are skills in information giving and using communication skills, such as open questions, listening skills and picking up on cues to encourage patients to share their agenda, beliefs and expectations about medicines (see chapter 3 for further information on consultation skills and decision making).

Such skills are important, but need to be used in conjunction with the prescriber's reflection on attitudes and beliefs about the purpose of the interaction, i.e. that what is required is for the healthcare professional to use skills that facilitate the overall goal of supporting patients and using opportunities to contribute to the decisions that they currently make about medication – decisions that fit with the patient's own preferences and personal circumstances. As the Medicines Partnership (2007) competencies indicate, this requires a non-judgemental attitude to patients and respect for their expertise and the decisions that they make about medicine taking.

Table 9.1 Examples of shared decision-making competencies (Medicines Partnership 2007)

Listening

Listens actively to the patient

Gives the patient the opportunity to express their views

Listens to the patient's views and discusses any concerns

Communicating

Helps the patient to interpret information in a way that is meaningful to them

Uses open questions to elicit information

Displays a non-judgemental attitude

Context

With the patient, defines and agrees the purpose of the consultation

Establishes how involved the patient wants to be in decisions about their treatment

Keeps focused on the agreed aims of the consultation

Knowledge

Has up-to-date knowledge of the area of practice and wider health services

Works in partnership with colleagues

Is aware of practical resources and aids to help the patient

Understanding

Recognises that the patient is an individual

Agrees goals with the patient

Respects the patient's knowledge and expertise regarding their own condition

Exploring

Discusses illness and treatment options, including no treatment

Elicits what the patient understands about their illness and treatment

Explores what the patient thinks about medicines in general

Discusses what the symptoms and/or illness may be caused by and how it can be managed

Establishes whether the health professional or patient have similar or different views about an illness and/or symptoms

Discusses any misunderstandings about illness and/or treatments

Encourages the patient to express positive and negative views about treatment/no treatment options

Deciding

Decides with the patient the best management strategy

Explains own thought processes and reasons why medicines may or may not be necessary

Provides full and accurate information about the pros and cons of all treatment options including any side effects

Discusses prognosis and likely health outcomes

Communicates uncertainty and risk to the patient

Checks that the patient understands reasons behind the decisions

Negotiates with the patient about the treatment decisions

Gives the patient time to consider the information before making a decision if appropriate

Accepts the patient's decisions

Table 9.1 (cont.)

Explores the patient's ability to undertake the agreed plan

Checks that the patient knows what they are taking and why

Monitoring

Agrees with the patient what happens next

Ensures that the patient knows what to do if their symptoms change or if a problem arises

Expresses a willingness to review the decision

It is also important to highlight that the skills and competencies of concordance will also often be used by nurses and other healthcare professionals within the context of an existing or ongoing relationship with a patient. This pattern of contact may well be different to that available to doctors, and this may therefore represent an opportunity for nurses, allied health professionals and pharmacists to improve on the often poor communication that has characterised doctors' prescribing interactions in the past, as demonstrated, for example, in Cox et al.'s (2003) systematic review (see below). Not only do nurses and allied health professionals often have ongoing relationships with their patients, they are also often valued by patients specifically for professional and personal characteristics, such as approachability and accessibility. This fact has also been highlighted in evaluations of nurse prescribing: Latter and Courtenay's (2004) review of literature on the effectiveness of nurse prescribing found that one of the key positive elements to emerge from the first wave of nurse prescribing in the UK was the value that patients placed on their relationship with their prescribing nurse. Nurses therefore need to exploit this in the interests of effective medicines management by ensuring that they are building on their relationships with patients where possible and are using the skills and competencies of concordance in the context of this valued relationship.

The skills and competencies outlined above also make it clear that concordance involves effective communication between members of the healthcare team and regular review of prescribed medicines, a requirement that is consistent with Government recommendations on supplementary prescribing.

The most recent development in guidelines for concordance in the UK is the establishment of national guidelines for medicines concordance by the National Institute for Clinical Excellence (NICE 2009).

Experienced healthcare professionals reading this will perhaps consider that they already practice concordance, that they have a holistic partnership approach to interactions, including those focused on medicines, as well as the communication skills required to put this approach into practice operationally. Often these principles and skills are perceived as 'second nature' and something that they have simply acquired as part of their clinical experience. However, the majority of research investigating nurses' and other healthcare professionals' approach to medicines interactions points to the conclusion that their interactions fall short of demonstrating concordance in practice. A review of this research and its implications for IPs and SPs is given below.

Concordance – what are healthcare professionals doing in practice?

While research into concordance in practice remains scarce to date, a review of the available evidence begins to shed light on current practice and enables some implications for prescribing nurses to be drawn from this.

A systematic review of research into communication between patients and healthcare professionals about medicine taking and prescribing has been undertaken by Cox et al. (2003). The aim of the review was to identify and summarise research on two-way communication between patients and healthcare professionals in order to inform the model of concordance. The review focused on 134 qualitative and quantitative studies published between 1991 and 2000 and included both intervention and non-intervention studies that spanned a variety of countries. Most of the studies examined elements of what is now known as concordance, even if the original studies did not define it as such – for example, research into 'encouraging patients to ask questions about medicines' and 'involving patients in discussions about medicines' is reviewed. Unsurprisingly, the majority of studies have focused on doctors' communication about medicines, with a minority also describing pharmacist and patient communication behaviours. Comparatively few studies in the review focus on nurses or allied health professionals, and this is perhaps not surprising given the relatively recent emergence of these professional groups internationally into the prescribing arena. However, valuable insights and lessons can be drawn from previous research into doctor and pharmacist communication behaviours with patients about their medicines.

From their review, Cox et al. (2003) conclude that 'much of the research indicated that communication between patients and professionals retains the asymmetry typical of paternalistic healthcare professional-patient interactions… Therefore the evidence examined in this review suggests that it is unlikely that concordance is taking place'. The authors do however note that there was evidence that it was possible to move towards a concordant approach in practice if certain preconditions were in place, such as doctors encouraging patient participation and listening attentively to their concerns. They also note that where some degree of concordance had taken place in practice, positive outcomes were noted, such as improved satisfaction and adherence. This therefore adds weight to the argument that nurses and other healthcare professionals should be striving for concordance in practice. The conclusions also point to the fact that healthcare professionals have some way to go to achieve it.

A more detailed analysis of Cox et al.'s review is beyond the scope of this chapter, but, in addition to the above overall conclusions, the review also highlights that patient preferences for participation and partnership in interactions and decision making are complex and dynamic. As with the research into the more general concept of patient participation, the research in Cox et al.'s review indicates that patients vary in the extent to which they wish to, for example, engage in discussion about medicines and share decisions about medicines management. It is likely that these preferences may be at least partly bound up with previous experiences and expectations about roles and relationships in healthcare interactions (Latter et al. 2000). That is, if a patient has not experienced a two-way communication process with a healthcare professional, then he or she may not know how empowered they would feel if given the opportunity to become involved.

Two studies focusing specifically on the role and practice of nurses and aspects of medicines management draw similar conclusions to Cox et al.'s (2003) review, and also help give further detail on how nurses are practising and what is required in order to progress towards a more concordant approach in practice. Latter et al.'s (2000) study into nurses' role in medication education found that nurses across a range of clinical settings were generally limiting their role in patient medication education to simple information about the name of the drug, its purpose and the time of administration. There was little patient involvement in decisions about medication and little evidence to suggest that nurses were using the skills of concordance in practice, or were indeed aware of the evidence base about what should be used in practice. Patients' preferences for a low level of detail about their medication were cited by nurses as an inhibiting factor, as well as lack of time available and high workload. Interactions were more consistent with the evidence on good practice where the organisation of care in a clinical setting facilitated a good nurse–client relationship and where the clinical area was nurse-led rather than care decisions determined by medical or organisational priorities. Similar findings emerged from Rycroft-Malone's (2002) study, which focused specifically on patient participation in nurse–patient interactions about medication using a variety of qualitative methods, including conversational analysis as a data analysis technique. She found that a range of conversational strategies was employed by nurses to initiate and control conversations and this inhibited patients' participation. Predominantly, nurses did not encourage patients to take part in concordance-type interactions by, for example, assessing health beliefs and facilitating participation in decision making. Rycroft-Malone did however find that there was a range in the extent to which the nurses in her study facilitated participation, and the extent to which they were able to do this was dependent on the power balance inherent in nurse–patient relationships; nurses' communication style, knowledge, skills and experience; patients' age, acuity of illness and level of knowledge; and the organisation and philosophy of care adopted in the clinical setting.

Our more recent research into nurses who are prescribing medicines (Latter et al. 2007) included an evaluation of the communication competencies that nurses were using in their consultations with patients. In the national survey we conducted, most nurses reported that they worked in partnership with patients: 99% agreed or strongly agreed that they (a) saw patients as partners in the consultation and (b) applied the principles of concordance. In case studies of practice, we then drew on the NPC (2001) communicating with patients competencies, and applied these to our observation of nurses' prescribing consultations. Findings are shown in Table 9.2.

Our findings highlighted that nurse prescribers were regularly giving patients a range of information about medicines. In the majority of instances, nurses gave clear instructions to patients on how to take the medicine, and they also checked the patients' understanding and commitment to their treatment. However, as Table 9.2 shows, our study revealed that not all

Table 9.2 Communicating with patients: competencies observed in nurse prescribers' consultations (Latter et al. 2007)

Item	Yes	No	Total
Gives clear instructions to the patient – how to take the medicine (dose, use and duration)	89% (n=105)	11% (n=13)	100% (n=118)
Gives clear instructions to the patient – possible side effects and action to take in event of side effects	48% (n=57)	52% (n=61)	100% (n=118)
Checks patient's understanding and commitment to their treatment	73% (n=86)	27% (n=32)	100% (n=118)
Explains the nature of the diagnosis/patient's condition to the patient and the rationale behind it	66% (n=78)	34% (n=40)	100% (n=118)
Explains the potential risks and benefits of the treatment options to the patient	39% (n=46)	61% (n=72)	100% (n=118)
Assists the patient in making an informed choice about the management of their health problem	45% (n=54)	55% (n=64)	100% (n=118)
Listens to and understands the patient's beliefs and expectations	64% (n=76)	36% (n=42)	100% (n=118)
Shows evidence of understanding the cultural, language and religious implications of prescribing	14% (n=17)	86% (n=101)	100% (n=118)

consultations involved listening to patient beliefs and expectations, and consultations were much less likely to include information on side effects and the risks and benefits of treatment options. We concluded that while there is some cause for optimism based on evidence of nurse prescribers communicating effectively about some dimensions of medicines in their prescribing consultations, there is also evidence to suggest that they have not fully adopted a concordance or shared decision-making model of communication. Importantly, there is further potential to increase the frequency and comprehensiveness with which nurses explore patient health beliefs about medicines in their prescribing consultations. Further research is required in this area.

Conclusion

In this chapter, the meaning of concordance has been presented, together with an examination of the underpinning evidence base for effective prescribing consultations. Concordance has been compared with the traditional approach of compliance in medicine taking, and the evidence base for the latter has been shown to be inadequate in a number of respects. Competencies needed to enact concordance in practice have been outlined. While these may *appear* to be skills that healthcare professionals are familiar with, a warning against complacency is given by an examination of the research in this area to date – which suggests that concordance is not yet a feature of healthcare professionals' medicine interactions with patients.

Further research is required into the quality and effectiveness of healthcare professional prescribing interactions, including interventions to help professionals shift their practice towards a concordance approach, and the impact of this on patient outcomes, such as their health and medicines beliefs, medicine-taking behaviour and health outcomes.

Concordance is advocated as a key competency for nurses, pharmacists and allied health professionals who are now the new generation of prescribers. To move towards its use in practice is likely to maximise the true potential that the extension of prescribing powers represents, by enhancing not only patient access to the prescription of medicines, but also their access to medicine encounters that will truly enhance their ability to manage their medicines for the benefit of their health and wellbeing.

References

Carter, S., Taylor, D., Levenson, R. (2003). *A Question of Choice – Compliance in Medicine Taking*. London: Medicines Partnership.

Cox, K., Stevenson, F., Britten, N. et al. (2003). *A Systematic Review of Communication between Patients and Healthcare Professionals about Medicine-taking and Prescribing*. London: Guy's, King's and St Thomas' Concordance Unit.

Department of Health (2000). *Pharmacy in the Future: Implementing the NHS Plan. A Programme for Pharmacy in the NHS*. London: Stationery Office.

Department of Health (2001). *The Expert Patient Programme*. London: Department of Health.

Department of Health (2008). *High Quality Care for All: NHS Next Stage Review Final Report*. London: Department of Health.

Haynes, R.B., Ackloo, E., Sahota, N. et al. (2008). *Interventions for Enhancing Medication Adherence*. Issue 4. Oxford: Cochrane Library.

Horne, R., Weinman, J., Barber, N. et al. (2005). *Concordance, adherence and compliance in medicine-taking*. Report for the National Co-ordinating Centre for NHS Service Delivery and Organisation R&D. London: NHS.

Latter, S., Courtenay, M. (2004). Effectiveness of nurse prescribing: a review of the literature. *Journal of Clinical Nursing 13*: 26–32.

Latter, S., Yerrell, P., Rycroft-Malone, J. et al. (2000). *Nursing and Medication Education;*

Concept Analysis Research for Curriculum and Practice Development. Research Reports Series no 15. London: English National Board for Nursing, Midwifery and Health Visiting.

Latter, S., Maben, J., Myall, M. et al. (2007). Perceptions and practice of concordance in nurses' prescribing consultations: findings from a national questionnaire survey and case studies of practice. *International Journal of Nursing Studies 44*(1): 9–18.

Marinker, M., Shaw, J. (2003). Not to be taken as directed: putting concordance for taking medicines into practice. *British Medical Journal 326*: 348–349.

Medicines Partnership (2003). *Project Evaluation Toolkit*. Keele: Medicines Partnership.

Medicines Partnership (2007). *A Competency Framework for Shared Decision-making With Patients* (first edition). Keele: Medicines Partnership Programme at NPC Plus.

National Institute for Health and Clinical Excellence (2009). *Medicines Adherence: Involving Patients in Decisions About Prescribed Medicines and Supporting Adherence. Clinical Guideline 76*. London: NICE.

National Prescribing Centre (2001). *An Outline Framework to Help Nurse Prescribers*. Liverpool: NHS National Prescribing Centre.

Pound, P., Britten, N., Morgan, M. et al. (2005). Resisting medicines: a synthesis of qualitative studies of medicine-taking. *Social Science and Medicine 61*(1): 133–155.

Royal Pharmaceutical Society of Great Britain (1997). *From Compliance to Concordance: Achieving Shared Goals in Medicine-taking*. London: Royal Pharmaceutical Society of Great Britain.

Rycroft-Malone, J. (2002). *Patient Participation in Nurse-patient Interactions About Medication*. Unpublished PhD thesis. Southampton: School of Nursing and Midwifery, University of Southampton.

Shaw, J.M., Mynors, G., Kelham, C. (2005). Information for patients on medicines. *British Medical Journal 331*: 1034–1035.

Vermeire, E., Hearnshaw, H., Van Royen, P. et al. (2001). Patient adherence to treatment: three decades of research. A comprehensive review. *Journal of Clinical Pharmacy and Therapeutics 26*: 331–342.

Vermeire, E., Wens, J., Van Royen, P. et al. (2005) *Interventions for Improving Adherence to Treatment Recommendations in People with Type 2 Diabetes Mellitus*. Issue 2. Oxford: Cochrane Library.

Evidence-based prescribing

Trudy Granby and Stephen R. Chapman

According to Sackett et al. (1996) evidence-based healthcare is: 'judiciously and conscientiously applying the best evidence to prevent, detect and treat disorders'.

This is an ambitious statement as the barriers to disseminating and applying evidence are both numerous and multifaceted.

The discipline of evidence-based medicine (EBM) is relatively new to nurses; traditionally they have based their clinical decisions on a combination of experience, observation, opinion, published material and personal research (Trinder and Reynolds 2000). The introduction of clinical governance, which emphasises accountability, quality and efficiency, has challenged this approach and it is no longer acceptable to base clinical decisions on personal opinion. Decision making must be evidence-based.

Prescribing is only one stage in making a rational treatment decision. Other stages include drawing on individual clinical expertise, taking account of patient choice and considering available resources. This needs to follow a 'step-wise' approach, starting with defining the patient's problem, which requires specific clinical skills and expertise, including undertaking a detailed history and physical examination, interpreting test results etc. In some circumstances, treatment may be initiated before a firm diagnosis has been made. In this situation, the clinician has to draw upon the best information available at the time and their knowledge of the patient.

It is essential that the patient is involved in making the treatment decisions. The patient's beliefs, expectations and preferences should be identified and acknowledged alongside existing clinical evidence. If a treatment is unacceptable to a patient, they are unlikely to adhere to the regime.

Evidence-based clinical practice is an approach to decision making. It is about considering, and then applying, the best evidence available when deciding how to treat an individual patient, groups of patients or populations (Gray 1997).

It is a structured process and requires the practitioner to be able to:

- Recognise and understand certain criteria, such as safety, effectiveness and efficacy.
- Access evidence and assess its quality.
- Recognise whether the results can be generalised and/or can be applied to the individual, group or population.

This chapter provides a brief insight into some of the issues surrounding evidence-based prescribing including clinical and cost effectiveness, hierarchy of evidence, recognising the benefits or harm of a treatment and concordance.

Some facts and figures

In England during 2008, drugs used to treat chronic conditions, such as cardiovascular disease, conditions of the central nervous system, respiratory disease and endocrine disorders, accounted for around 60.5% of the total items dispensed from NHS prescriptions in the community (http://www.ic.nhs.uk/).

Prescribing, supplying and administering medicines is now probably the most common healthcare intervention. In England during 2007, 796 million items were dispensed from NHS prescriptions in the community, 88.6% of which were free to patients, at a net ingredient cost £8372.7 billion. On average, 15.6 items were dispensed per head of population. (http://www.ic.nhs.uk/). To give a comparison, an increase of 49.5% in real terms over 1997.

In the acute healthcare sector, during 2007 medicines accounted for over 25.7% of the total cost of overall NHS expenditure on medicines, i.e. £11.2 billion (http://www.ic.nhs.uk/). Around £90 million worth of medicine is taken into hospitals every year by patients – most of these are destroyed. 7000 individual doses of medication are administered in a 'typical' hospital every day and administration of medicines takes up approximately 40% of nurses' time (Audit Commission 2001).

It could be assumed that this massive spending on medicines has resulted in an improvement in the health of the population. Although most patients do benefit from the medicines they are prescribed, this is not always the case; 50% of patients with chronic conditions fail to take their medication as prescribed (DoH 2000a). Since the introduction of the Yellow Card scheme in 1964 more than 40 000 suspected adverse reactions to drugs have been reported to the Committee on Safety of Medicines (CSM)/Medicines and Healthcare products Regulatory Agency (MHRA). Around 17% of older inpatients, experience an adverse drug reaction (Audit Commission 2001) and medication errors cost the NHS around £500 million each year in additional inpatient days. Furthermore, around 25% of clinical negligence cases stem from hospital medication errors (DoH 2000b).

How can we improve things?

The main focus of the NHS reforms (DoH 2000c) is to improve the quality of care received by patients by increased access to the services required and the medicines required to treat their illness. One way in which this can be achieved is to extend the roles of some healthcare professionals enabling them to prescribe, supply and administer medicines. If prescribing is to be effective, the practitioner must be able to:

- Identify the problem in terms of the patient's (or population's) needs and the ultimate goal of any treatment.
- Break the problem down into more explicit questions, such as, 'What are the treatment options? How well do they work? What are the resource implications?'
- Check the evidence.

In order to do this, the following must be considered:

How effective are the treatment options?

To answer the above, two issues must be considered – *efficacy and clinical effectiveness*. They are quite different.

Efficacy is when a drug is proven to have a pharmacological effect greater than a placebo. This does not necessarily translate into an improved clinical outcome.

Clinical effectiveness is when that efficacy results in a proven clinical outcome.

For instance, if Drug A lowers blood pressure by 2 mm mercury it has proven clinical efficacy, and could, in theory get a licence. If, however, using Drug A to lower blood pressure by 2 mm mercury has no effect on the desired outcome (that is it doesn't have any effect on stroke preven-tion) then it is not clinically effective.

This is an important differentiation. A drug can be efficacious, and have a licence, but may not be the drug of choice when clinical outcome (that is effectiveness) is considered. In other words, just because it has a licence it isn't necessarily the optimal drug.

Is the drug cost effective?

In a publicly-funded cash limited health economy, such as a Primary Care Trust, making sure that a drug represents value for money is as much a part of evidence-based prescribing as clinical effectiveness. It is particularly important to rationalise one's thinking around *marginal benefit.*

This is best illustrated by the following example, outlined in Box 1, of two hypothetical drugs used to treat the common cold – Drug A and Drug B.

Box 1 An illustration of marginal costs and benefits

Drug A cures colds completely in 90% of cases
Drug B cures colds completely in 80% of cases
Drug A costs £10
Drug B costs £5
You have £1000 to treat patients in your PCT
Drug A treats £1000/10 × 90% = 90 patients
Drug B treats £1000/5 × 80% = 160 patients

In this example, you can treat almost twice the number of patients to cure by using a less effective drug. If, however, you had a cold, and you could afford it, you may prefer to pay the extra £5 to cure your cold. Thus you are applying different values when using public money – this tension exists in making all prescribing decisions – having to balance the needs of the individual against the needs of the population.

This active dynamic is illustrated in an article by Barber (1995). He represents this dia-grammatically (see Figure 10.1) adding the dimension of patient choice to Parish's (1973, cited in Barber, 1995) original definition of appropriateness, safety, effectiveness and cost.

Health economies and organisations, such as The National Institute of Clinical Excel-lence (NICE), which seek to balance costs and benefits, use health economic modelling. These models are often complex and sophisticated. While prescribers do not need a detailed knowledge of health economies, it does help to have a basic understanding of the key terms.

In the simplest form, if two drugs have the same clinical effect, then it makes sense to prescribe the cheapest alternative – this is known as *cost-minimisation.*

Cost-effective analysis is one method by which the cost of treatment can be compared with expected outcome, for example, reduction in blood pressure. Effectiveness is measured in natural units, such as drop in millimetres of mercury.

Cost-benefit analysis takes this a stage further by allocating a cost to the differences in these natural units. The conventional way of carrying out cost-effectiveness analysis involves con-sidering additional costs over and above the cost of the medicine. These include **direct costs**

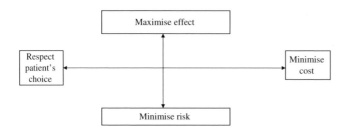

Figure 10.1 Aims of good prescribing – and their commonest conflicts (Barber 1995)

(the cost of the medicine, staff time involved in carrying out the therapy, equipment required to do this and any costs to the patient, e.g. transport to clinics); **indirect costs** (how time spent by staff could have been otherwise used); and **intangible costs** (such as pain and adverse effects) (Phillips and Thompson 1997).

For example, in a hospital the intravenous anaesthetic Propofol is more expensive per unit than conventional general anaesthetic which means that the direct costs are higher. However, using Propofol means that patients have fewer side effects and recover more quickly from the effects of the anaesthetic which speeds up discharge from hospital. This, in turn, results in more surgical procedures being performed as day cases, thus avoiding the 'hotel costs' of overnight accommodation in hospital. Avoiding these direct costs makes Propofol more cost effective. Health economic studies need to be examined as carefully as clinical trials and should be critically appraised before rushing to conclusions – Drummond et al.'s paper and that of the Evidence–based Medicine Working Group give an excellent guide to key points to check (Drummond 1997; O'Brien 1997). There is also an easy to read, light hearted look at a 'crooks guide' on how pharmacoeconomic studies are designed to ensure drugs look expenditure-effective in the book *Pharmacoeconomics* (Wally et al. 2004)

Checking the evidence

The evidence available to support prescribing decisions can be derived from a number of sources.

- Published evidence.
- Personal experience.
- Reasoning and intuition.
- Colleagues and peers.
- Promotional material.

If an effective prescribing decision is to be made, attention to the published evidence is crucial. Published evidence varies in terms of quality and credibility. Studies can therefore be ranked according to a 'hierarchy of evidence' (see Table 10.1).

Systematic reviews and/or meta-analysis

Good quality systematic reviews provide the best indication of the effects of an intervention. These reviews use a robust, formalised process to summarise available research evidence (Egger et al. 2001). By asking a number of therapeutic questions, e.g. the intention of the therapy, the patient group and the outcome of the intervention, this process identifies those studies that warrant inclusion in the review. The results of studies reviewed are then combined (using meta-analysis) to assess the effectiveness of the intervention. Issues such as the quality

Table 10.1 Hierarchy of evidence (Jones 2002)

I. Systematic reviews and Meta-analysis

II. Randomised controlled double blind trials

III. Cohort studies

IV. Case control studies

V. Cross-sectional surveys

VI. Case series

VII. Case reports

of the studies included and the possibility and likely impact of bias and chance are discussed to help contextualise the review.

Systematic reviews are often published in leading journals and can also be accessed via a range of websites (see Table 10.2 at the end of this chapter for further details). The Cochrane website is a particularly good independent source for such reviews.

Meta-analysis is a technique used to combine study findings. This form of analysis is most frequently used to assess the effectiveness of a therapeutic intervention by combing data of two or more randomised controlled trials. The findings of trials involving large numbers are generally more reliable. Combining the results in this way provides an estimate of the effects of a particular intervention. However, it must be remembered that any meta-analysis is dependent on the quality of the individual studies. With this in mind, prescribers need to be able to appraise studies and interpret the findings for themselves or, alternatively, check with independent reviews, such as Cochrane.

Randomised controlled trials are normally used to assess the effects of a particular drug. Typically, two groups are studied: one group receives the intervention; while the other group acts as the control. Patients are allocated to study groups randomly by a 'process analogous to flipping a coin' to avoid bias. This type of study can be developed further by setting up systems to ensure that neither the researcher nor the patient is aware of who is receiving the intervention. This is known as 'double-blinding.'

Cohort studies are often used to find out what causes a particular disease. Subjects with a specific disease, or who have certain characteristics, are identified and followed-up over a period of time to monitor progress and/or detect complications. For instance, the Framingham study has charted the progress of heart disease, stroke and other conditions in a cohort of American men over 50 years. (see www.framingham.com/heart). Cohort studies are often done retrospectively from large databases, such as the General Practice Research database, which have historical data.

Case control studies examine the causes of a disease. In these studies, a group of patients with a particular disease are compared to a group with similar characteristics (such as age, sex and concurrent medical conditions) but who don't have the disease. Case control studies compare histories of those in the group to identify any exposure to possible causal factors.

Cross-sectional surveys measure the frequency of a disease or risk factor in a defined group, at a given time. These surveys can be used to determine the prevalence of a condition.

Case reports are descriptive, anecdotal reports of the medical history of one patient. A *case series* is a collection of similar reports. As there is no control group, case reports and case series are not statistically valid. However, they are useful in alerting others of rare occurrences or the emergence of 'new' diseases.

Table 10.2 Some sources of information available from the Internet

Peer reviewed journals

Annals of Internal Medicine	www.annals.org
British Medical Journal (BMJ)	www.bmj.com
Journal of the American Medical Association (JAMA)	www.jama.ama-assn.org
New England Journal of Medicine	www.nejm.org
The Lancet	www.thelancet.com

Systematic Reviews and Digests of Reviews

Aggressive Research Intelligence Facility (ARIF)	www.bham.ac.uk/arif
Bandolier	www.jr2.ox.ac.uk/bandolier
Clinical Evidence	www.clinicalevidence.com
Cochrane Library	www.nelh.nhs.uk/cochrane.asp
Database of Abstracts of Reviews of Effectiveness (DARE)	www.york.ac.uk/inst/crd/darehp.htm
Drugs and Therapeutics Bulletin	www.dtb.org.uk/dtb/index.html
Effective Health Care Bulletins	www.york.ac.uk/inst/crd/ehcb.htm
Effectiveness Matters	www.york.ac.uk/inst/crd/em.htm
Evidence-based Medicine	ebm.bmjjournals.com/
Health Technology Assessment	www.york.ac.uk/inst/crd/htahp.htm
MeReC Bulletins, Briefings and Extras	www.npc.co.uk
NHS Centre for Reviews and Dissemination Reports	www.york.ac.uk/inst/crd/crdrep.htm
NHS Economic Evaluation Database (NHS EED)	www.york.ac.uk/inst/crd/nhsdhp.htm

Research in Progress

National Research Register	www.doh.gov.uk/research/nrr.htm

Guidance

eGuidelines	www.eguidelines.co.uk
Midland Therapeutic Review and Advisory Committee (MTRAC)	www.keele.ac.uk/depts/mm/MTRAC/
National Institute for Clinical Excellence	www.nice.org.uk
PRODIGY	www.prodigy.nhs.uk
Scottish Intercollegiate Guidelines Network (SIGN)	www.sign.ac.uk/

Other resources

British National Formulary	www.bnf.org
Centre for Evidence-based Medicine	www.cebm.net/
DrugInfoZone	www.druginfozone.org
Electronic Medicines Compendium	emc.medicines.org.uk
Medicines Partnership	www.medicines-partnership.org
National electronic Library for Health	www.nelh.nhs.uk
National Prescribing Centre	www.npc.co.uk
National Service Frameworks	www.doh.gov.uk/nsf/nsfhome.htm
Netting the Evidence	www.nettingtheevidence.org.uk

Table 10.2 (cont.)

NPC Current Awareness Bulletin (eCAB)	www.npc.co.uk/ecab/ecab.jsp
UK Medicines Information	www.ukmi.nhs.uk
Virtual Health Network	www.vhn.net

Recognising the benefits or harms of a treatment

In order to decide whether a drug should be prescribed, it is useful to know whether intervening with that drug in an experimental group produced a different effect to intervening with a placebo (that is an identical looking tablet or capsule with no active ingredient) in a control group. The results of such trials allow us to estimate the probability of a greater benefit, and/or, what are the risks of harmful outcomes, such as side effects. Benefits and harms are presented in a number of ways, which can affect how they are perceived (Bucher et al. 1994). It is therefore important to have an understanding of what these terms mean, as well as the principles underpinning them.

Results are often presented in terms of reducing risk, either as absolute risk reduction or relative risk reduction. Reporting relative risk reduction, tends to show an increased positive effect. Absolute and relative risks are sometimes reported within the same paper. It is important to have an understanding of the differences between the two.

Absolute risk

The absolute risk is the chance of developing a condition, for example, the risk of contracting an infection may be 1 in 100 000.

Relative risk

The relative risk is the chance of developing a condition when a factor is present, divided by the risk of developing the condition when that factor is absent. For instance, if 20 out of a 100 patients develop a skin rash when taking a drug, whereas only 5 out of a 100 get a skin rash when taking a placebo, the relative risk is 20/100 divided by 5/100, which is 4. In other words, the risk of developing a rash when taking that drug is 4 times greater than when not taking the drug.

Caution needs to be taken when examining at relative risk, as it takes no account of background incidence. It should, therefore, always be considered in the context of absolute risk. For example, if the absolute risk of infection is 1 in 100 000, and the relative risk is 2, the risk increases to 2 in 100 000, which is still very low. However, if the absolute risk of infection is 1 in 5, and the relative risk is 2, the risk increases by 2 in 5 – an increase of 20%, which would probably be unacceptable.

Absolute risk reduction (ARR)

Absolute risk reduction is the absolute amount by which an intervention can reduce the absolute risk. This is calculated as:

ARR = (event rate in the control group – event rate in the intervention group) × 100

(Sackett 2000)

To illustrate this, suppose 2000 people received Drug X (*the intervention group*) and 2000 people received a placebo – *the control group*. The *intention* is to prevent death.

In the intervention group, 360 people died making the event rate 360/2000. In the control group, 500 people died, making the event rate 500/2000.

So, applying the above calculation, the ARR is (**500 – 360)/2000 × 100 that is 140/2000 × 100**, a reduction in the death rate of 7%.

Relative risk reduction (RRR)

RRR reports how much a risk is reduced by an intervention as a comparative percentage of the control. This is calculated by dividing the difference between the rate of events in the control and intervention groups by the rate of events in the control group. So, if we relate back to the example used to calculate the ARR, the RRR is (**360/2000**) – (**500/2000)/500/2000 *that is* 0.07/0.25**, a reduction in death rate of 28%.

Number needed to treat (NNT)

This is probably the most useful way of expressing results as it tells the prescriber how many patients, with a given condition, they need to treat with a particular intervention, before one additional patient benefits. To use Moore and McQuay's (1997) example, let's suppose that 100 people are given an analgesic. Of these, 70 people have their pain relieved within 2 hours. However, when these same 100 people are given a placebo instead of the analgesia, only 20 have their pain relieved within 2 hours. We can assume that the pain was relieved by the analgesia in 50 **(70–20)** cases. This is an absolute risk reduction of **(70/100 – 20/100) i.e. 0.5.**

The NNT is calculated by dividing 1 by the ARR, that is 1/(control event rate – experimental event rate), in this case 1/0.5, which gives an NNT of 2. This means that 2 people have to take the analgesic for one of them to obtain relief as a result of taking that analgesic. This is a very low NNT, which means it is an optimal treatment. Although there is no cut-off point, once NNTs go over 100 (that is over 100 patients have to be treated by a drug for 1 patient to benefit), prescribers should be more circumspect.

Odds ratios

The odds of an event happening are calculated by taking the number of times something happens and dividing that by the number of times it doesn't happen. For example, let's say that for every 100 people buying a raffle ticket, 26 win something (the event happens) and 74 don't (the event doesn't happen). To work out the odds of winning, 26 is divided by 74, making the chance of winning 0.35 **i.e. 35%**. Any number over 1 means that the chances of winning are good, anything below 1 means that the chances of winning are unlikely.

However, knowing the odds is not enough when deciding whether a drug intervention is effective – this involves knowing whether there is a difference between the odds of something happening to the group receiving a particular intervention, and the control group who don't receive the intervention. This is known as the ***odds ratio***, which is calculated by dividing the odds in the treatment group with the odds in the control group.

For example, Drug A, is believed to cure the common cold within 24 hours of the first symptoms appearing. It is given to 100 people and works in 60 cases. Therefore, the odds of this happening in this group are 60/40, which is 1.5. Placebo A is given to another 100 people with the same symptoms. This time 20 people recover in 24 hours, making the odds 20/80, which is 0.25. So, the odds ratio between the 2 groups is 1.5/0.25, that is 6.

As 6 is a much higher number than 1, the odds ratio suggests that Drug A is effective and thus worth prescribing. To explain this a little further, if 60 or more people from the placebo group had recovered, the odds ratio would have been 1 or less. This would have shown that the drug had an effect equivalent to, or less than a placebo, and would not be worth prescribing.

Obviously, this is a very simplistic example. In reality, calculating event rates, reported as odds ratios, is not that easy and some would argue against describing the effects of treatments in this way. However, odds ratios are frequently used. This is possibly because they provide a way of presenting benefit (or harm) within a wide range of values: zero to infinity.

Further examples of risk reductions, odds ratios etc. are given in Trisha Greenhalgh's book *How to Read a Paper: The Basics of Evidence Based Medicine* (2006).

Guidelines

The increase in the amount of available information has, paradoxically, increased the risk of unacceptable variations in the way certain conditions are managed. In order to manage this risk, organisations have produced guidelines (at both national and local levels) to help stand-ardise best practice. Providing these guidelines are robust, reliable, and properly implemented, they are really useful when making prescribing decisions and should improve healthcare by reducing the variations. However, applying guidelines to individuals still requires some degree of judgement, as no recommendation can take into account the many varied circumstances of an individual.

Guidelines are used in a range of ways to promote effective and efficient care. Locally developed guidelines should encompass valid, national guidelines, such as NICE guidance, and should be prioritised to address local need. Some sources of guidelines are listed in the table at the end of this chapter.

Finding the evidence

Keeping up-to-date with the amount of evidence can be very daunting. In order to make good use of the often limited time available, it should help to know how to keep up-to-date by knowing which journals should be used and where to find independent reviews of the evidence.

The internet possibly offers the easiest, and most effective route to keeping up-to-date, and many websites operate an email alert service. Some of these websites are password protected and require a subscription to access full text. However, they do usually allow access to abstracts. However, the internet is not without its hazards as anyone can post information on it. Using a standard search engine to look for information may lead to sponsored sites, which may carry an element of bias or have incomplete information. With this is mind, it is advisable to always check whom the site is sponsored by, and ideally restrict your searches to the sites we have listed below.

Will the patient follow the treatment?

Regardless of the evidence, a medicine can only be effective if the patient follows the treatment regime. There are many, and often complicated reasons why a patient fails to do this. In some cases this may be related to the cost of 'cashing in' the prescription (Jones and Britten 1998). But even when patients have access to their medicine, they don't always follow the prescribers' instructions. This may reflect the clinicians' approach to consultation (see chapter 3 consultation skills and decision making), whereby the patient does not have the opportunity to discuss any concerns (Barry et al. 2000). Indeed, how the consultation is conducted is a cornerstone to the concept of concordance, which is based on the prescriber and patient working together, as equals, to form a 'concord' that is, a contract or, if you prefer, a therapeutic alliance. The aim of this therapeutic alliance is to create a situation whereby the patient feels able to share the decision making around the management of their condition, including which medicines are prescribed (RPSGB1998).

To help make this happen, the prescriber must ensure that the patient has an understanding of their condition and is aware of all of the treatment options, including the associated risks and benefits. This approach is quite the opposite to the prescriber dominated, paternalistic approach associated with compliance whereby the prescriber makes these decisions and instructs the patient on what they should do.

Concordance may present the prescriber with some challenges. By increasing the patient's knowledge about treatment options and inviting them to make decisions about which treatment they would prefer, the patient may not choose what the prescriber considers to be the best option. Furthermore, there may be times when a patient refuses drug intervention (for example, they may feel the risk of unwanted side effects outweighs the potential benefits of taking the drug). While this may feel uncomfortable to some clinicians, it does demonstrate concordant behaviour as the patient is demonstrating that they have understood the options, yet exercised their right to refuse the treatment.

Is the concordant approach more effective in terms of ensuring better use of medicines and increasing patient outcomes than other approaches? As yet, concordance has not been extensively evaluated. However, a recent systematic review of the literature related to concordance found that two-way communication between patients and professionals resulted in several benefits, including increased adherence to treatment regimens, increased health outcomes and fewer medication-related problems (Cox et al. 2003). See chapter 9 (Promoting concordance in prescribing interactions: the evidence) for a fuller discussion of the work by Cox et al. and an overview of the evidence base for the concept of concordance.

To conclude, if prescribers are to realise the full potential of their role, they must base their prescribing decisions on the best available evidence. For this to happen they need to create ways to ensure they keep abreast of any new evidence relating to their area of clinical practice. By doing so they will ensure that their patients receive safe, effective treatment and also equip themselves with the knowledge, confidence and competency to fully contribute to the development and delivery of a modernising National Health Service.

References

Audit Commission (2001). *A spoonful of sugar: medicines management in NHS hospitals.* London: Audit Commission.

Barber, N. (1995). What constitutes good prescribing? *British Medical Journal 310*: 923–925.

Barry, C.A. et al. (2000). Patients unvoiced agenda in general practice consultations: Qualitative study. *British Medical Journal 320*: 1246–1250.

Bucher, H.C., Weinbacher, M. et al. (1994). Influence of method of reporting study results on decision of physicians to prescribe drugs to lower cholesterol concentration. *British Medical Journal 309*: 761–764.

Committee on Safety of Medicines/Medicines and Healthcare products Regulatory Agency.

Monitoring the safety and quality of medicines: The Yellow Card Scheme. See http://medicines.mhra.gov.uk

Cox, K., et al. (2003). *A systematic review of communication between patients and health care professionals about medicine-taking and prescribing.* London: GKT Concordance Unit. King's College

Department of Health (2000a). *Pharmacy in the future: implementing the NHS plan. A programme for pharmacy in the National Health Service.* London: Stationery Office

Department of Health (2000b). *Organisation with a memory.* London: Stationery Office

Department of Health (2000c). *The NHS Plan: A plan for investment, A plan for reform.* London: Stationery Office.

Drummond, M.F. et al. (1997). How to use an article on economic analysis of clinical practice A. Are the results of the study valid? *Users' guides to the medical literature. JAMA 277*: 1552–1557.

Egger, M. et al. (2001). *Systematic reviews in health care: meta-analysis in context.* London: BMJ Publishing Group.

Framingham study. See www.framingham.com/heart.

Gray, J.M. (1997). *Evidence-based healthcare.* Edinburgh: Churchill Livingstone.

Greenhalgh, T. (2006). *How to read a paper: the basics of evidence based medicine* (third edition). London: BMJ books.

Jones, C. (2002). Research Methods (1). *The Pharmaceutical Journal 268*: 839–841.

Jones, I., Britten, N. (1998). Why do some patients not cash in their prescriptions? *British Journal of General Practice 48*: 903–905.

Moore, A., McQuay, H. (1997). *What is an NNT?* Hayward Medical Communications Ltd.

O'Brien, B. et al. (1997). How to use an article on economic analysis of clinical practice B. What are the results and will they help me in caring for patients? Users' guides to the medical literature. *JAMA 277*: 1802–1806.

Parish, P.A. (1973). Drug prescribing- the concern of all. Journal of the Royal Society of Health. Cited in: Barber, N. (1995). What constitutes good prescribing? *British Medical Journal 310*: 923–925.

Philips, C. Thompson, G. (1997). *What is cost-effectiveness?* Hayward Medical Communications Ltd.

Royal Pharmaceutical Society of Great Britain (1998). *From compliance to concordance: achieving shared goals in medicines taking.* London: Royal Pharmaceutical Society.

Sackett, D.L., Rosenburg, W.M.C. et al. (1996). Evidence based medicine: what it is and what it isn't. *British Medical Journal 312*: 71–72.

Trinder, L., Reynolds, S. (eds) (2000). *Evidence-based Practice: A critical appraisal.* Oxford: Blackwell Publishing.

Wally, T. et al. (eds) (2004). *Pharmacoeconomics.* Churchill Livingstone.

Extended/supplementary prescribing: a public health perspective

Sarah J. O'Brien

In this chapter we consider the wider, public health context of independent/supplementary prescribing.

Public health

Public health is defined as 'the science and art of preventing disease, prolonging life, and promoting health through the organised efforts of society' (Acheson 1988). Public health professionals must consider health and disease in the widest possible context and take action to promote healthy lifestyles, prevent disease, protect and improve general health, and improve healthcare services (FPH 2009). Thus public health practice is focused on enhancing the health of the population as a whole, rather than necessarily treating individual patients. The definition of 'population' varies with context. This may be geographical (e.g. a locality like a general practice population), or in terms of particular client groups (e.g. children or people on low incomes) or people with specific health needs (e.g. people with diabetes or heart disease).

Public health personnel, working with other professional groups, fulfil a number of functions and, broadly speaking, their work usually falls within one or all of the following three domains: improving health; protecting health; and improving health services (FPH 2009). The work includes monitoring the health status of the population, identifying health needs, building programmes to reduce risk and screen for early disease, controlling and preventing communicable diseases, developing policies to promote health, planning and evaluating healthcare provision, and managing and implementing change (Chief Medical Officer 2003a).

Although delivering good health for the population is generally considered to involve more than simply prescribing medicines, two recent therapeutics-based public health interventions have been launched. The first is the widespread use of statins for reducing the risk of coronary events (Ward et al. 2007) and the second is over-the-counter sales of orlistat for managing overweight and obese individuals (Idelevich et al. 2009; Lancet 2009). However, the debate continues surrounding the possible long-term consequences of such measures (Goldstein et al. 2009; Lancet 2009). Where medication is needed, it is important to be familiar with the policies that guide prescribing in a public health context.

Patients and society

Prescribed medicines are the most frequently supplied treatments for NHS patients. The total drugs budget in the financial year 2006/07 was approximately £10.6 billion, of which approximately £7.6 billion was spent in primary care and £3 billion in hospital care. In 2006 alone some 752 million prescription items were dispensed in the community (DoH 2008a). In considering the impact of extended/supplementary prescribing there is a balance to be struck between the benefits that it may afford for the individual patient and the effects on the population. In essence, therefore, prescribing decisions should benefit the individual without being detrimental to society as a whole. This is exemplified in the sphere of antimicrobial prescribing. Using antibiotics in one patient may influence the efficacy and efficiency of that antibiotic for use in another patient through the development of resistance. So the needs of an individual must be balanced against the necessity to preserve the value of antimicrobial agents for the community as a whole. It should also be borne in mind that the societal impact of profligate use of antimicrobials might affect the treatment options for future generations.

Widening access to antimicrobials

Supplementary prescribing, community practitioners, nurse prescribing, nurse and pharmacist independent prescribing and patient group directions have all served to widen the range of healthcare professionals, other than doctors and dentists, who can now prescribe antimicrobials (Reeves 2007). According to NHS Prescription Services (2009), penicillins accounted for the majority of nurse prescribing in 2008/09 (7.8% of some 11.6 million items prescribed by nurses).

In addition to the regulated means of gaining access to antimicrobials, individuals with access to the internet have the potential to purchase medicines, including antimicrobials, by mail order. This poses risks to patients and prescribers alike. Not only may patients self-medicate inappropriately, with all the inherent dangers of ineffective treatment, masking infections or serious adverse drug reactions, but they may fail to declare to a prescriber any medication that they have acquired by this route. This emphasises the importance of asking explicitly about over-the-counter or over-the-internet purchases as part of clinical history taking.

Policies on antimicrobial prescribing

Antimicrobial agents are used to treat infections in individual patients and in public health interventions to control disease outbreaks (Tapsall 2003). Policies on antimicrobial prescribing are directed towards limiting the development and further spread of antimicrobial resistance. But rationalising antimicrobial use is a complex issue, requiring commitment from clinicians, professional societies, the public, the Government and international agencies (Keuleyan and Gould 2001).

Antimicrobial resistance

The public health importance of antimicrobial resistance remains the subject of much concern, debate and study. The emergence of antimicrobial resistance has, by and large, been correlated with the rise and fall of specific antimicrobial use in medical practice. For example, in Finland, after nationwide reductions in the use of macrolide antibiotics for outpatient therapy, there was a significant decline in the frequency of erythromycin resistance among Group A streptococci isolated from throat swabs and pus samples (Seppälä et al. 1997). It is generally agreed, however, that the use of antimicrobials in veterinary clinical practice and in agriculture has also played a part in promoting resistance in organisms that infect humans (Tollefson and Karp 2004), although the debate continues (Wassenaar 2005). As early as 1969, the Swann Committee recommended that certain antibacterial agents should only be prescribed for veterinary use and should not be used as growth promoters (Anon. 1969). However, attempting to reverse the effects of antibiotic selection pressure by withdrawal of the substance is complex and resistance determinants may persist at low, but detectable, levels for many years in the absence of the corresponding drugs (Johnsen et al. 2009). In Sweden antibiotic use for outpatients decreased from 15.7 defined daily doses per 1000 inhabitants per day in 1995 to 12.6 defined daily doses per 1000 inhabitants per day in 2004 as a result of a concerted campaign to curb the spread of antibiotic-resistant clones of *Streptococcus pneumoniae* (Mölstad et al. 2008). Although epidemic spread of a penicillin-resistant pneumococcal clone across southern Sweden was halted, the national prevalence rose from 4% to 6% during the same period.

Such is the weight attached to the public health problems posed by antimicrobial resistance that the announcement of nurse prescribing in 2001 prompted a debate in the House of Lords (UK Parliament 2002).

The term antimicrobial agent encompasses antibacterial, antifungal, antiprotozoal and antiviral agents. Although the term is often used synonymously to mean 'antibiotic', in fact antibiotics form a subset of antimicrobial agents. Antimicrobial agents eradicate susceptible organisms but problems arise because of the resistant organisms that survive to infect other individuals. The development of antimicrobial resistance is a straightforward example of natural selection, i.e. 'the survival of the fittest' (SMAC 1998). Resistance can arise through spontaneous, random genetic mutations, through transfer of resistance genes between organisms or through the selection of inherently resistant species. The importance of these processes varies with organisms, antimicrobial agents and clinical situations. A description of the mechanisms of antimicrobial resistance is given in the Standing Medical Advisory Committee's (SMAC) report *The Path of Least Resistance* (1998). Multi-resistance occurs when an organism is resistant to two or more unrelated antimicrobial agents. There is much evidence in the peer-reviewed literature of antimicrobial resistance in many organisms. However, what is much less clear is which parameters of antibiotic consumption promote resistance (Reeves 2007).

Resistant organisms that continue to cause concern, or have emerged in recent years, include:

- Meticillin-resistant *Staphylococcus aureus* (MRSA) – a cause of bacteraemia in patients in healthcare settings (Johnson et al. 2005).
- Multi-drug resistant tuberculosis (MDR-TB).
- Extended spectrum beta-lactamase-producing *Escherichia coli* (ESBL *E. coli*) – an increasingly recognised cause of urinary tract infections in patients in hospital and the community (Livermore et al. 2007).
- Panton-Valentine leucocidin (PVL)-positive *Staphylococcus aureus* and MRSA causing skin and soft-tissue infections and life-threatening invasive infections, such as necrotising pneumonia and necrotising fasciitis (O'Brien et al. 2004; Zetola et al. 2005).
- Ciprofloxacin-resistant *Enterobacteriaceae* causing a variety of food-related illnesses (Cattoir and Nordmann 2009; Parry and Threlfall 2008).
- Multi-drug resistant bacteria *Pseudomonas aeruginosa* in cystic fibrosis patients (Health Protection Agency 2008; Woodford and Ellington 2007).
- Vancomycin-resistant staphylococci and enterococci (Leclercq 2009).
- Glycopeptide-resistant enterococci causing bacteraemia (Fisher and Phillips 2009).

Consequences of antimicrobial resistance

Most anxiety tends to be concentrated on resistance to antibacterial agents, although it should be borne in mind that similar issues are emerging with antifungal and antiviral agents, particularly resistance to antivirals for treating Human Immunodeficiency Virus (HIV) (Alteri et al. 2009) and influenza (Jonges et al. 2009; Weinstock and Zuccotti 2009). There are several consequences of antimicrobial resistance. Firstly, it may make infections more difficult to treat and treatment failures across a range of infections, and in a variety of settings, have been documented (Davey and Marwick, 2008). Treatment failures, at best, necessitate the use of alternative drugs, which are often more expensive and may have unwelcome side effects (SMAC 1998). In the case of resistant tuberculosis, incomplete treatment or treatment failures can also have direct public health implications in terms of onward transmission of a resistant organism to others in the community (Kan et al. 2008; Schmid et al. 2008).

Secondly, the infection may be more severe. For example, there was a significant excess of deaths in Danish patients infected with antimicrobial drug-resistant *Salmonella typhimurium* (Helms et al. 2002) and in patients in the UK with MRSA (Delaney et al. 2008). There is also evidence that infection with a resistant organism leads to a longer duration of illness (Helms et al. 2002) or greater length of hospital stay (Lee et al. 2006; Sunenshine et al. 2007). Increases in treatment and associated costs also occur (Cosgrove 2006; Maragakis et al. 2008; Nicolau 2009).

In summary, antimicrobial resistance can adversely affect patient outcome by enhancing virulence, causing a delay in administering appropriate therapy and limiting available therapy (Cosgrove and Carmeli 2003).

Controlling antimicrobial resistance

If antimicrobials are viewed as a valuable public resource then a societal goal must be to minimise resistance (McGowan 2001). Indeed, the control of antimicrobial resistance is a major Government priority, guided by two very influential expert reports, *The Path of Least Resistance* from the SMAC Sub-group on Antimicrobial Resistance (1998) and *Resistance to Antibiotics and Other Antimicrobial Agents* from the House of Lords Select Committee on Science and Technology (1998), both of which expressed major concerns about the increasing clinical and public health importance of antimicrobial resistance. In 2000 the Department of Health issued its *UK Antimicrobial Resistance Strategy and Action Plan* (2000). This was followed shortly thereafter by a complementary plan in Scotland (Scottish Government 2002).

The main aims of the Government's strategy are to reduce morbidity and mortality of infections due to antimicrobial resistant organisms and to maintain the effectiveness of antimicrobial agents in the treatment and prevention of infections in animals and man (DOH 2000). There are three interconnected elements – surveillance, prudent antimicrobial use and infection control, underpinned by improvements in information technology and a co-ordinated research programme.

Surveillance

Surveillance is essential in controlling antimicrobial resistance, as has been amply demonstrated in Scandinavia (Mölstad et al. 2008) and the UK (Health Protection Agency 2008). For individual patients, and where clinical samples have been submitted for laboratory investigation, information from susceptibility testing allows informed decisions on the best therapeutic options. When the information from each individual report is collated centrally (in England by the Health Protection Agency, in Wales by the National Public Health Service and in Scotland by Health Protection Scotland), monitoring changing resistance patterns may indicate emerging problems, leading to appropriately targeted interventions and control measures. Knowledge gleaned from surveillance data concerning prevailing antimicrobial resistance patterns should also inform the development of prescribing policies (for both hospitals and the community), and thus guide empirical prescribing.

In 2008 the Health Protection Agency published the fifth in a series of reports on antimicrobial resistance in England, Wales and Northern Ireland (Health Protection Agency 2008). The authors noted the continued decline in the proportion of *Staphylococcus aureus* bacteraemias attributable to MRSA (from 38% in 2006, to 31% in 2007). They noted that meningococci remained susceptible to the first line antimicrobial agents (penicillin, cefotaxime, rifampicin and ciprofloxacin) that are used for treatment and chemoprophylaxis. They reported that while resistance to ciprofloxacin in *Escherichia coli* causing bacteraemia had plateaued between 2006 and 2007, the rise of resistance in *Shigella* spp. isolates to nalidixic acid and ciprofloxacin, as well as the emergence of resistance to third-generation cephalosporins, was increasingly limiting treatment options. Finally they highlighted the first appearance in 2007 of high-level azithromycin resistance in *Neisseria gonorrhoeae* (although azithromycin is not recommended for treatment of gonorrhoea, it is widely used in *Chlamydia trachomatis* infection) and the unexpected emergence of oseltamivir-resistant influenza viruses that was subsequently confirmed as a problem worldwide.

The data presented by the Health Protection Agency illustrate the value of antimicrobial susceptibility testing in informing antimicrobial prescribing. Susceptibility patterns for many pathogens, especially respiratory tract pathogens, may change over short distances, making local medical microbiology services essential for rational prescribing decisions (SMAC 1998). Medical microbiologists can advise on appropriate specimen collection and there are often local protocols providing guidance on the types of specimens that need to be obtained in particular clinical situations, including the timing in relation to transport to the laboratory. Knowledge of local resistance patterns gained through diagnostic testing then helps to guide local antimicrobial prescribing policies. It is incumbent on prescribers to familiarise themselves with local antimicrobial resistance patterns and local antimicrobial prescribing policies. All Trusts and Primary Care Trusts are required to implement and review local policies and guidelines on appropriate antimicrobial use on an annual basis. In the SMAC report (1998) it was noted that guidelines should be evidence-based, including the strength of that evidence, and bear the date on which they were developed. They should contain information on the agent, dosage, frequency and length of course. Finally they should indicate where local policy varies from national advice.

As well as understanding what is happening to microorganisms with respect to antimicrobial resistance, there is also a need for better data on antimicrobial usage in the UK and to correlate better information on antimicrobial usage patterns, trends in antimicrobial resistance and clinical disease in both the human and animal populations due to antimicrobial-resistant organisms. For the first time in 2008 the Health Protection Agency report contained data on antimicrobial prescribing. Since there is a broad consensus that a major driver of antimicrobial resistance is the use (particularly overuse and misuse) of antimicrobial agents, surveillance of antimicrobial prescribing is important for a better understanding of the epidemiology of antimicrobial resistance. Tighter controls on the use of antimicrobials in both medical and veterinary clinical practice are welcome and are already well underway in the UK. However, agricultural and clinical practice (both veterinary and medical) elsewhere in the world will continue to have an impact on resistant bacteria identified in the UK through foreign travel and global trade.

Controlling healthcare associated infections (HCAIs) goes hand in hand with curbing antimicrobial resistance. Two key documents that have served to shape policy to control HCAIs are *Winning Ways* (Chief Medical Officer 2003b) and *Towards Cleaner Hospitals and Lower Rates of Infection* (DoH 2004a). The increased focus on control of HCAIs led to the introduction in the NHS of mandatory surveillance for *Staphylococcus aureus* (MRSA) bacter-aemia in April 2001, glycopeptide-resistant enterococcal bacteraemia in October 2003 and *Clostridium difficile* associated disease in January 2004.

Prudent antimicrobial prescribing

The Clinical Prescribing Subgroup of the Interdepartmental Steering Group on Resistance to Antibiotics and Other Antimicrobial Agents, in its report *Optimising the Clinical Use of Anti-microbials: Report and Recommendations for Further Work* (2001), defined prudent antimi-crobial prescribing as:

> The use of antimicrobials in the most appropriate way for the treatment or preven-tion of human infectious diseases, having regard to the diagnosis (or presumed diagnosis), evidence of clinical effectiveness, likely benefits, safety, cost (in com-parison with alternative choices), and propensity for the emergence of resistance. The most appropriate way implies that the choice, route, dose, frequency and duration of administration have been rigorously determined.

They considered that prudent meant *both* 'less' (they deemed that there was still scope to reduce unnecessary use of antimicrobials) *and* 'appropriate' (i.e. the right dose of the right antibiotic, administered via the most appropriate route for the right length of time to produce a clinical cure, while minimising side effects and the development of resistance).

A number of ways to optimise antimicrobial prescribing in clinical practice has been developed. In its report *The Path of Least Resistance*, the SMAC (1998) published 'four things you can do'. These were:

> No prescribing of antibiotics for simple coughs and colds.
>
> No prescribing of antibiotics for viral sore throats.
>
> Limit prescribing for uncomplicated cystitis to three days in otherwise fit women.
>
> Limit prescribing of antibiotics over the telephone to exceptional cases.

The majority (around 80%) of antimicrobial prescribing takes place in primary care and approximately half of these prescriptions are issued for respiratory tract infections. Yet the evidence that there are benefits from prescribing antibiotics for sore throats (Del Mar et al. 2006), sinusitis (Small et al. 2007) and acute otitis media (Thanaviratananich et al. 2008; Vouloumanou et al. 2009) is fairly limited. In certain circumstances, empirical therapy for a range of infections may be justified, but this also illustrates the importance of carefully evalu-ating symptoms and employing appropriate diagnostic tests (NICE 2007; 2008). A useful resource for guiding diagnosis and management is the NHS Clinical Knowledge Summaries, available at http://www.cks.nhs.uk/home. NHS Evidence comprises a compilation of the best available evidence, available at www.evidence.nhs.uk. Its principal aim is to improve health and patient care by providing easy access to a comprehensive evidence base for everyone in health and social care taking decisions about treatments or the use of resources (including clinicians, public health professionals, commissioners and service managers). It builds on the significant international reputation of the National Institute for Health and Clinical Excellence for developing high-quality evidence-based guidance (http://www.nice.org.uk).

Management of infection guidelines for primary care, which can be adopted for local use, have been developed by the Association of Medical Microbiologists and the Health Protection Agency and are available at http://www.hpa.org.uk/web/HPAwebFile/HPAweb_C/1194947340160. Another important consideration for the nurse or pharmacist prescriber is to appreciate when a patient may benefit from a medical opinion. This is analogous to the situation when a GP may seek the help of a specialist hospital colleague.

In a survey by Kumar and colleagues (2003), GPs who were prescribing antibiotics for sore throat were found to be unsure which patients were likely to benefit from antibiotics. They tended to prescribe for patients who they judged to be more unwell or those from more deprived backgrounds because of fears about complications. They were also more likely to prescribe in pressurised clinical situations. Similarly, Mangione-Smith and colleagues (2006) found that when parent questioned a treatment plan it increased physicians' perceptions that antibiotics were expected, in turn leading to increased inappropriate antibiotic prescribing. However, the encouraging news is that antimicrobial prescribing policies can change clinicians' behaviour (Arnold and Straus 2005; Davey et al. 2005) although the precise interventions can be many and varied. It has been suggested that multidisciplinary approaches including participation from physicians, nurses, pharmacists and infection control staff are successful (Gross and Pujat 2001; Pflomm 2002; Saizy-Callaert et al. 2003). However, while alterations in prescribing behaviour have been observed, the evidence that this has yet had an effect on antimicrobial resistance is more limited (Reeves 2007).

In addition to ensuring that professionals are enabled to prescribe antimicrobials optimally in clinical practice, the Government's strategy also includes provision of better diagnostic and antimicrobial susceptibility testing methods, providing more rapid information to prescribers, while safeguarding surveillance data.

Another key component of the strategy is managing public expectations. This recognises that patients, too, have a role in reducing antimicrobial resistance by not expecting inappropriate treatment (Holmes et al. 2003). Macfarlane and colleagues (1997a) provided a graphic illustration of this. They surveyed 1014 patients who had recently consulted their GP with an acute lower respiratory tract infection. Of the 787 patients who replied to the questionnaire, 656 of the 662 patients who attributed their symptoms to an infection thought that antibiotics would help. Moreover, 564 patients wanted an antibiotic, 561 expected to receive one and 146 actually requested one. In an internet-based questionnaire study conducted in the Netherlands, 44.6% of 935 survey participants accurately identified antibiotics as being effective against bacteria and not viruses. Nearly 60% of respondents considered that acute bronchitis required treatment with antibiotics. The perceived need for antibiotics for respiratory tract infection-related symptoms ranged from 6.5% for cough with transparent phlegm, to 46.2% for a cough lasting for more than two weeks (Cals et al. 2007). Mangione-Smith and colleagues (2004) have also demonstrated significant racial and ethnic differences in parents' expectations for antibiotics.

In the SMAC report (1998), attention was drawn to the need for a public campaign to handle patients' expectations and to influence their attitudes towards antimicrobial agents. First launched in 2002, the Department of Health re-ran its national public information campaign during 2008 and 2009 to remind the public that antibiotics are ineffective in treating viral infections, such as colds, most coughs and sore throats. (DoH 2002; 2009). Evidence shows that where patients are involved in decision making about their care, coupled with better information about their condition and the advantages and disadvantages of antimicrobial therapy, access to and completion of appropriate antimicrobial therapy is improved (Davey et al. 2002). Re-consultation rates may also go down (Macfarlane et al. 1997b).

Infection control

This part of the Government's strategy is aimed at reducing the spread of infection in general (and hence limiting the need for using antimicrobial agents) and of antimicrobial resistant organisms in particular. The costs of nosocomial infections (Kilgore et al. 2008; Stone et al. 2005) and bloodstream infections are substantial (Kilgore and Brossette 2008). In a large hospital survey in the UK, it was estimated that around 8% of inpatients presented with one or more hospital-acquired infections during the inpatient period (Plowman et al. 2001). The estimated costs of these infections to the hospital sector were in the region of £930 million. In a national point prevalence survey of HCAIs in Scotland between October 2005 and October 2006, the prevalence was 9.5% in acute hospitals and 7.3% in non-acute hospitals. The highest prevalences of HCAIs in acute hospital inpatients were in care of the elderly (11.9%), surgery (11.2%), medicine (9.6%) and orthopaedics (9.2%). The lowest prevalence occured in obstetrics (0.9%) (Reilly et al. 2008). Similar prevalence rates have also been reported in Finland (Lyytikäinen et al. 2005).

Despite the importance of HCAIs, it seems that they have not always been afforded the priority by the NHS that they deserve. In his report *Winning Ways – Working Together to Reduce Healthcare Associated Infection in England,* the Chief Medical Officer (2003b) reaffirmed commitment to tackling this intractable problem. He outlined the need for senior management commitment, local infrastructure and systems, making it clear that dealing with HCAIs must not be left to clinical staff alone. Each organisation providing NHS services now has a Director of Infection Prevention and Control who, among other things, oversees and implements local infection control policies, is responsible for the Infection Control Team and reports directly to the Chief Executive and the Board. Importantly, they have the authority to challenge inappropriate clinical hygiene, as well as antimicrobial prescribing decisions, and they are an integral member of the organisation's clinical governance and patient safety groups. A public annual report must also be produced. One of the seven action areas in the Chief Medical Officer's report related to high standards of hygiene in clinical practice. Updated guidelines for preventing HCAIs were published by Pratt et al. (2007) and are also available at the 'epic' (evidence-based practice in infection control) website at http://www.epic.tvu.ac.uk/PDF Files/epic2/epic2-final.pdf.

Prudent antimicrobial prescribing in hospitals was also referred to in *Winning Ways* (Chief Medical Officer 2003b), with the development of the hospital pharmacy initiative (DoH 2003a), and illustrates how closely intertwined are the dual themes of prudent prescribing and infection control.

The Government is concerned to strengthen infection control practices not only in hospitals but also in the community. This is in recognition of the fact that there are more beds in the community, with patients staying in them for longer, than in hospital, coupled with increasing numbers of nursing and residential homes and hospices. The volume and types of surgical procedures being carried out in primary care are increasing and the shorter hospital stays enabled by minimally invasive surgery mean that infections previously detected and dealt with in hospital are now being identified and managed in the community. The National Institute for Health and Clinical Excellence (NICE) (2003) published detailed guidelines on preventing HCAIs in primary and community care in 2003. These were developed by Thames Valley University under the sponsorship of the National Collaborating Centre for Nursing and Supportive Care (Pellowe et al. 2003).

Developmental standards proposed by the Government in its document *Standards for Better Health* (DOH 2004b) included that healthcare be provided by well-designed environments that are appropriate for safe and effective delivery of treatment, care or specific functions, including effective control of HCAIs. The Care Quality Commission (http://www.cqc.org.uk) is responsible for developing detailed criteria underpinning these standards and for inspecting NHS delivery and performance against all core and developmental standards. This high-profile approach is indicative of the priority afforded to infection control.

Notifiable and other communicable diseases

Under the Public Health (Control of Disease) Act 1984 and the Public Health (Infectious Diseases) Regulations 1988, certain infectious diseases are notifiable by law. Under current legislation the legal duty to notify rests with a doctor. It follows, therefore, that medical colleagues need to be informed of any diseases required to be notified to the Proper Officer of the local authority, which is usually a Consultant in Communicable Disease Control in the local health protection unit. Notification forms are available from the local authority and a fee is payable for each notification. The Public Health (Control of Disease) Act 1984 requires that the following information is disclosed: the patient's name; age; sex; and address. The legal duty to notify these personal details has not been superseded by the Data Protection Act (McTigue and Williams 2003). Notification should take place on clinical suspicion that a patient is suffering from a notifiable disease. It need not await laboratory confirmation. Indeed, the delays inherent in obtaining a laboratory diagnosis might mean that secondary spread has already occurred.

The list of notifiable diseases, which can found in the *British National Formulary*, includes food poisoning. In 1992, the Advisory Committee on the Microbiological Safety of Food defined food poisoning as any condition of an infectious or toxic nature, caused by or thought to be caused by contaminated food or water (ACMSF 1992). Although treatment, other than supportive measures, is not usually recommended for patients with uncomplicated gastroenteritis, symptoms may herald an outbreak of food poisoning. Useful advice on when to contact the local Consultant in Communicable Disease Control is contained in the Communicable Disease Control Handbook (Hawker et al. 2005).

The purpose of notification is to allow the Proper Officer to take prompt public health action and institute control measures as soon as possible, within the incubation period of the disease in question, in order to prevent more people from becoming unwell. These control measures may include vaccination.

Vaccination policy

The childhood vaccination programme represents one of the most successful public health interventions of modern times. Diseases like poliomyelitis and diphtheria, which were still major child killers as late as the 1950s, are now virtually eliminated. In May 1980, less than 200 years after Edward Jenner demonstrated that vaccination with material from cowpox protected against the development of smallpox, the World Health Assembly accepted that smallpox had been eradicated from the world (Fenner 1993). Now, ironically, concerns arise from its potential use as a bioterrorist agent.

The aims of vaccination programmes are to achieve herd immunity in the susceptible population against those diseases which are spread from person to person, e.g. measles, and to protect everyone against infections from other sources, e.g. tetanus (Hawker et al. 2005). These aims are met either through inducing active immunity, through the use of inactivated or live attenuated organisms or their products, or through inducing passive immunity by means of immunoglobulins. Active immunity is long-lasting, whereas passive immunity, although offering immediate protection, is short-lived. Some of the considerations in offering vaccinations are outlined below, but detailed guidance is available on the Department of Health website at http://www.dh.gov.uk/en/Publichealth/Healthprotection/Immunisation/Greenbook/DH_4097254, where updated chapters from the 'Green Book' on *Immunisation Against Infectious Disease* (Department of Health et al. 2006) are posted from time to time. The replacement chapters represent current Department of Health recommendations and should be followed in place of the 2006 version. Communications from the Chief Medical Officer or the Chief Nursing Officer regarding vaccination should be kept on file for future reference.

Consent for vaccination

Consent must always be obtained before vaccinating a child and parents must always feel that they have been fully included in the decision. Consent is needed at the time of each immunisation, after the child has been judged to be a suitable candidate including being fit enough to receive the vaccine (Department of Health et al. 2006). Consent that has been obtained before the child has been brought in to receive the vaccine is an agreement for the child to be included in the programme. Consent should still be sought for the vaccination to be given, and written consent provides a permanent record.

Vaccines: storage, distribution and disposal

Detailed instructions can be found in the 'Green Book' in chapter 3. In essence, vaccines should be stored according to the manufacturer's instructions. They should be kept on the shelves in a designated vaccine refrigerator, the temperature of which can be constantly monitored. Careful attention should be paid to the shelf life, so that vaccines that have reached their expiry date are not used, and written procedures for storage, distribution and disposal of vaccines should be audited regularly.

Vaccines: indications and contraindications

There are some conditions that increase the risk of complications from an infectious disease, and people with these conditions should be immunised as a priority (Department of Health et al. 2006). These conditions include asthma, chronic lung disease, congenital heart disease, Down's syndrome, HIV infection, small for dates babies and babies born prematurely. People with no spleen, or who have functional hyposplenism, are at increased risk from certain bacterial infections, like *Streptococcus pneumoniae*, and should receive appropriate cover. Haemodialysis patients are at increased risk of hepatitis B and hepatitis C, and, following vaccination, their hepatitis B markers should be monitored regularly and re-immunisation offered as needed.

General contraindications to vaccination include an acute febrile illness and a definite history of a severe local or general reaction to a preceding dose of a vaccine. Where there is doubt about what might constitute a severe local or general reaction, advice can be sought from clinical colleagues like a Consultant Paediatrician, Consultant in Communicable Disease Control or the District Immunisation Co-ordinator. Definitions of severe local and general reactions to vaccination are given in chapter 8 of the 'Green Book'.

It is not advisable to give live virus vaccines to pregnant women because of the theoretical possibility of harming the foetus. However, where there is a significant risk that a pregnant woman has been exposed to a disease, like poliomyelitis or yellow fever, the indications for vaccination outweigh the potential risk to the foetus. Administration of live virus vaccines is also contraindicated in certain groups of patients with impaired immunity, e.g. those undergoing treatment for malignancy, recent bone marrow transplant recipients, those on high dose steroids or other immunosuppressants and people with impaired cell-mediated immunity like those with HIV infection. There are specific contraindications to individual vaccines and all those prepared to administer vaccines should ensure that they have read the most up-to-date information from the manufacturer and have studied the relevant chapters in the 'Green Book', checking for updates on the Department of Health website.

Vaccination procedures

Covered in-depth in chapter 4 of the 'Green Book', a major consideration is that, before administering any vaccine, the individual should have received training and be proficient in the appropriate techniques including subcutaneous, intramuscular and intradermal injection techniques. The individual must have made appropriate arrangements for dealing with anaphylactic shock (see 'Green Book' chapter 8) and other immediate reactions. The person administering the vaccine should have familiarised themselves with the procedures when they need to give more than one vaccine at the same time. Those performing vaccinations should also know about and understand the procedures for reporting adverse reactions through the 'Yellow Card' scheme to the Medicines Control Agency.

The childhood vaccination programme

The current immunisation schedule is as follows (Department of Health et al. 2006):
   For neonates: BCG and hepatitis B vaccinations may be indicated for certain groups.
   For children:

When to immunise	What to give
Two months old	Diphtheria, tetanus, pertussis (whooping cough), polio and *Haemophilus influenzae* type b (Hib) (DTaP/IPV/Hib)
Pneumococcal (PCV)	
Three months old	Diphtheria, tetanus, pertussis (whooping cough), polio, Hib (DTaP/IPV/Hib) and meningococcal serogroup C (MenC)
Four months old	Diphtheria, tetanus, pertussis (whooping cough), polio Hib (DTaP/IPV/Hib), MenC and PCV
12 months old	Hib/MenC
Around 13 months old	Measles, mumps and rubella (MMR), PCV
Three years four months to five years old	Diphtheria, tetanus, pertussis and polio (DTaP/IPV or dTaP/IPV), Measles, mumps and rubella (MMR)
12 to 13 years (girls only)	Human papillomavirus (HPV)
13 to 18 years old	Tetanus, diphtheria and polio (Td/IPV)

Adapted from Department of Health et al. 2006 (chapter 11)

For adults: booster doses of tetanus and polio, if appropriate, and vaccines for lifestyle/occupational risks.

For adults over 65 years: a single dose of pneumococcal polysaccharide vaccine, if they have not previously received it, and annual influenza vaccination.

Influenza and pneumococcal vaccines may be recommended at any age for special medical risk groups, and vaccines offering protection for overseas travel may also be indicated at any age (although some have a lower age limit).

The UK immunisation schedule changes from time to time, on advice from an independent expert advisory committee, the Joint Committee on Vaccination and Immunisation. For example, the most recent addition to the schedule is human papillomavirus (HPV) vaccination, which is routinely recommended for all girls at 12 to 13 years of age (school year 8, or S2 in Scotland, or school year 9 in Northern Ireland) (DOH 2008b).

Protecting the health of travellers overseas

In 2001 the Department of Health published the second edition of the sister companion to the 'Green Book' (Department of Health et al. 2001). *Health Information for Overseas Travel*, or the 'Yellow Book' as it has become known, is a concise and authoritative source of information about the common health risks faced by overseas travellers and the ways to reduce them. Like the 'Green Book' it is also available through the Department of Health website at http://www.archive.official-documents.co.uk/document/doh/hinfo/travel02.htm. The National Travel Health Network and Centre (NaTHNaC) is also a very useful source of advice and up-to-date health information for overseas travel (http://www.nathnac.org).

Final thoughts

Implementing independent/supplementary prescribing is intended to benefit individual patients and society as a whole. Although much of this chapter has focused on antimicrobial resistance and vaccination, the principles outlined with regard to prudent prescribing apply equally well to drugs other than antimicrobials. *Building on the Best* (DOH 2003b) extended patient choice through a number of measures, including easier availability of repeat prescriptions and extending the range of over-the-counter medicines that will be available for purchase without a prescription. Thus prescribers also need to be alert to the fact that patients might have obtained other medicines over the counter and that these might interact with prescribed medication. And in McTigue's (2004) useful summary on managing clinical risks she provides some practical suggestions for managing the risks associated with repeat prescribing.

References

Acheson, E.D. (1988). *Public Health in England: Report of the Committee of Inquiry into the Future Development of the Public Health Function*. London: Department of Health.

Advisory Committee on the Microbiological Safety of Food (1992).

Alteri, C., Svicher, V., Gori, C. et al. Study Group S (2009). Characterisation of the patterns of drug resistance mutations in newly diagnosed HIV-1 infected patients naive to the antiretroviral drugs. *BMC Infect Dis* 9(1): 111.

Anon. (1969). *Report of the Joint Committee on the Use of Antimicrobials in Animal Husbandry and Veterinary Medicine (Swann Committee)*. London: HMSO.

Arnold, S.R., Straus, S.E. (2005). Interventions to improve antibiotic prescribing practices in ambulatory care. *Cochrane Database Syst Rev* (4): CD003539.

Cals, J.W., Boumans, D., Lardinois, R.J. et al. (2007). Public beliefs on antibiotics and respiratory tract infections: an internet-based questionnaire study. *Br J Gen Pract* 57(545): 942–947.

Cattoir, V., Nordmann, P. (2009). Plasmid-mediated quinolone resistance in gram-negative bacterial species: an update. *Curr Med Chem* 16(8): 1028–1046.

Chief Medical Officer (2003a). *Public Health in England*. http://www.dh.gov.uk/en/Aboutus /MinistersandDepartmentLeaders/ChiefMe dicalOfficer/Archive/FeaturesArchive/Brow sable/DH_4102835 (accessed 22 July 2009).

Chief Medical Officer (2003b). *Winning Ways – Working Together to Reduce Healthcare Associated Infection in England. A Report from the Chief Medical Officer*. London: Department of Health.

Cosgrove, S.E. (2006). The relationship between antimicrobial resistance and patient outcomes: mortality, length of hospital stay, and health care costs. *Clin Infect Dis 42* (Suppl. 2): S82–S89.

Cosgrove, S.E., Carmeli, Y. (2003). The impact of antimicrobial resistance on health and economic outcomes. *Clin Infect Dis 36*: 1433–1437.

Davey, P.G., Marwick, C. (2008). Appropriate vs. inappropriate antimicrobial therapy. *Clin Microbiol Infect 14* (Suppl. 3): 15–21.

Davey, P., Pagliari, C., Hayes, A. (2002). The patient's role in the spread and control of bacterial resistance to antibiotics. *Clin Microbiol Infect 8* (Suppl 2): 43–68.

Davey, P., Brown, E., Fenelon, L. et al. (2005). Interventions to improve antibiotic prescribing practices for hospital inpatients. *Cochrane Database Syst Rev* (4): CD003543.

Delaney, J.A., Schneider-Lindner, V., Brassard, P. et al. (2008). Mortality after infection with methicillin-resistant *Staphylococcus aureus* (MRSA) diagnosed in the community. *BMC Med 6*: 2.

Del Mar, C.B., Glasziou, P.P., Spinks, A.B. (2006). Antibiotics for sore throat. *Cochrane Database Syst Rev* (4): CD000023.

Department of Health (2000). *UK Antimicrobial Resistance Strategy and Action Plan*. London: Department of Health. http:// www.dh.gov.uk/en/Publicationsandstatistics /Publications/PublicationsPolicyAndGuida nce/DH_4007783 (accessed 22 July 2009).

Department of Health (2002). *Antibiotics – Don't Wear Me Out*. http://www.dh.gov.uk/ en/Publicationsandstatistics/Publications/Pu blicationsPolicyAndGuidance/DH_4007460 (accessed 28 July 2009).

Department of Health (2003a). *Hospital Pharmacy Initiative for Promoting Prudent Use of Antibiotics in Hospitals*. London: Department of Health. (Professional Letter. Chief Medical Officer: PLCMO (2003)3.) http: //www.dh.gov.uk/en/Publicationsandstatistics/ Lettersandcirculars/Professionalletters/Chief medicalofficerletters/DH_4004614 (accessed 29 July 2009).

Department of Health (2003b). *Building on the Best – Choice, Responsiveness and Equity in the NHS. A Summary*. London: Department of Health.

Department of Health (2004a). *Towards Cleaner Hospitals and Lower Rates of Infection: a Summary of Action*. London: Department of Health. http://www.dh.gov. uk/en/Publichealth/Healthprotection/Healt hcareacquiredinfection/Healthcareacquired generalinformation/index.htm (accessed 28 July 2009).

Department of Health (2004b). *Standards for Better Health – Health Care Standards for Services Under the NHS. A Consultation*. London: Department of Health.

Department of Health (2008a). *Pharmacy in England: Building on Strengths – Delivering the Future*. London: TSO (Cm 7341).

Department of Health (2008b). The 'Green Book' chapter on human papillomavirus (HPV). http://www.dh.gov.uk/en/Publicheal th/Healthprotection/Immunisation/Green book/DH_4097254. (accessed 29 July 2009).

Department of Health, National Assembly for Wales, Scottish Executive Health Department, DHSS PS (Northern Ireland), Public Health Laboratory Service Communicable Disease Surveillance Centre (2001). *Health Information for Overseas Travel*. London: The Stationery Office (also known as the 'Yellow Book').

Department of Health, Welsh Office, Scottish Office Department of Health, DHSS

(Northern Ireland). (2006. *Immunisation Against Infectious Disease* (eds Salisbury, D., Ramsay, M., Noakes, K.). London: HMSO (also known as the 'Green Book').

Department of Health (2009). Antibiotic campaign 2008–2009. Available at http://www.dh.gov.uk/en/Publichealth/Patientsafety/Antibioticresistance/DH_082512 (accessed 8th February 2010).

Faculty of Public Health (2009). *Public Health – Specialise in the 'Bigger Picture'*. http://www.fph.org.uk/careers/assets/files/ph_careers_booklet.pdf (accessed 8th February 2010).

Fenner, F. (1993). Smallpox: emergence, global spread, and eradication. *Hist Philos Life Sci* 15(3): 397–420.

Fisher, K., Phillips, C. (2009). The ecology, epidemiology and virulence of Enterococcus. *Microbiology* 155(Pt 6): 1749–1757.

Goldstein, M.R., Mascitelli, L., Pezzetta, F. (2009). Primary prevention of cardiovascular disease with statins: cautionary notes. *QJM* 102(11): 817–820.

Gross, P.A., Pujat, D. (2001). Implementing practice guidelines for appropriate antimicrobial usage: a systematic review. *Med Care* 39 (Suppl. 2): II55–II69.

Hawker, J., Begg, N., Blair, I. et al. (2005). *Communicable Disease Control Handbook (second edition)*. Oxford: Blackwell Sciences.

Health Protection Agency (2008). *Antimicrobial Resistance and Prescribing in England, Wales and Northern Ireland, 2008*. http://www.hpa.org.uk/web/HPAwebFile/HPAweb_C/1216798080469 (accessed 22 July 2009).

Helms, M., Vastrup, P., Gerner-Smidt, P. et al. (2002). Excess mortality associated with antimicrobial drug-resistant *Salmonella* typhimurium. *Emerg Infect Dis* 8: 490–495.

Holmes, J.H., Metlay, J., Holmes, W.C. et al. (2003). Developing a patient intervention to reduce antibiotic overuse. *Proc AMIA Symp* 2003: 864.

House of Lords Select Committee on Science and Technology (1998). *Resistance to Antibiotics and Other Antimicrobial Agents.*

7th Report 1997–98, HL Paper 81. London: Stationery Office.

Idelevich, E., Kirch, W., Schindler, C. (2009). Current pharmacotherapeutic concepts for the treatment of obesity in adults. *Ther Adv Cardiovasc Dis* 3(1): 75–90.

Interdepartmental Steering Group on Resistance to Antibiotics and Other Antimicrobial Agents (2001). Clinical Prescribing Subgroup. *Optimising the Clinical Use of Antimicrobials: Report and Recommendations for Further Work*. London: Department of Health. http://www.dh.gov.uk/prod_consum_dh/groups/dh_digitalassets/@dh/@en/documents/digitalasset/dh_4084395.pdf (accessed 29 July 2009).

Johnsen, P.J., Townsend, J.P., Bøhn, T. et al. (2009). Factors affecting the reversal of antimicrobial-drug resistance. *Lancet Infect Dis* 9(6): 357–364.

Johnson, A.P., Pearson, A., Duckworth, G. (2005). Surveillance and epidemiology of MRSA bacteraemia in the UK. *J Antimicrob Chemother* 56(3): 455–462.

Jonges, M., van der Lubben, I.M., Dijkstra, F. et al. (2009). Dynamics of antiviral-resistant influenza viruses in the Netherlands, 2005–2008. *Antiviral Res* 83(3): 290–297.

Kan, B., Berggren, I., Ghebremichael, S. et al. (2008). Extensive transmission of an isoniazid-resistant strain of Mycobacterium tuberculosis in Sweden. *Int J Tuberc Lung Dis* 12(2): 199–204.

Keuleyan, E., Gould, M. (2001). Key issues in developing antibiotic policies: from an institutional level to Europe-wide. European Study Group on Antibiotic Policy (ESGAP), Subgroup III. *Clin Microbiol Infect* 7 (Suppl 6): 16–21.

Kilgore, M., Brossette, S. (2008). Cost of bloodstream infections. *Am J Infect Control* 36(10): S172.e1–3.

Kilgore, M.L., Ghosh, K., Beavers, C.M. et al. (2008). The costs of nosocomial infections. *Med Care* 46(1): 101–104.

Kumar, S., Little, P., Britten, N. (2003). Why do General Practitioners prescribe antibiotics for sore throat? Grounded theory interview study. *BMJ* 326: 138.

Lancet (2009). Over-the-counter medicines: in whose best interests? *Lancet 373*(9661): 354.

Leclercq, R. (2009). Epidemiological and resistance issues in multidrug-resistant staphylococci and enterococci. *Clin Microbiol Infect 15*(3): 224–231.

Lee, S.Y., Kotapati, S., Kuti, J.L. et al. (2006). Impact of extended-spectrum beta-lactamase-producing *Escherichia coli* and *Klebsiella* species on clinical outcomes and hospital costs: a matched cohort study. *Infect Control Hosp Epidemiol 27*(11): 1226–1232.

Livermore, D.M., Canton, R., Gniadkowski, M. et al. (2007). CTX-M: changing the face of ESBLs in Europe. *J Antimicrob Chemother 59*: 165–174.

Lyytikäinen, O., Kanerva, M., Agthe, N. et al. (2005). Finnish Prevalence Survey Study Group. 2008. Healthcare-associated infections in Finnish acute care hospitals: a national prevalence survey. *J Hosp Infect 69*(3): 288–294.

Macfarlane, J., Holmes, W., Macfarlane, R. et al. (1997a). Influence of patients' expectations on antibiotic management of acute lower respiratory tract illness in general practice: questionnaire study. *BMJ 315*: 1211–1214.

Macfarlane, J.T., Holmes, W.F., Macfarlane, R.M. (1997b). Reducing reconsultations for acute lower respiratory tract illness with an information leaflet: a randomised controlled study of patients in primary care. *Br J Gen Pract 47*: 719–722.

Mangione-Smith, R., Elliott, M.N., Stivers, T. et al. (2004). Racial/ethnic variation in parent expectations for antibiotics: implications for public health campaigns. *Pediatrics 113*(5): e385–e94.

Mangione-Smith, R., Elliott, M.N., Stivers, T, et al. (2006). Ruling out the need for antibiotics: are we sending the right message? *Arch Pediatr Adolesc Med 160*(9): 945–952.

Maragakis, L.L., Perencevich, E.N., Cosgrove, S.E. (2008). Clinical and economic burden of antimicrobial resistance. *Expert Rev Anti Infect Ther 6*(5): 751–763.

McGowan, J.E. Jr. (2001). Economic impact of antimicrobial resistance. *Emerg Infect Dis 7*: 286–292.

McTigue, A. (2004). Taking stock: risk and remedy. *MPS Casebook 12*(1): 8–10. http://www.medicalprotection.org/uk/casebook/february2004 (accessed 28 July 2009).

McTigue, A., Williams, S. (2003). Have confidence in confidence alone. *MPS Casebook 11*(4): 8–10. http://www.medicalprotection.org/uk/casebook/november2003 (accessed 29 July 2009).

Mölstad, S., Erntell, M., Hanberger, H. et al. (2008). Sustained reduction of antibiotic use and low bacterial resistance: 10-year follow-up of the Swedish Strama programme. *Lancet Infect Dis 8*(2): 125–132.

NHS Prescription Services (2009). *Update on Growth in Prescription Volume and Cost in the Year to March 2009.* http://www.nhsbsa.nhs.uk/PrescriptionServices/Documents/Volume_and_cost_year_to_March_2009.pdf (accessed 23 July 2009).

NICE (2003). *NICE Clinical Guideline 2. Infection Control: Prevention of Healthcare-Associated Infection in Primary and Community Care.* http://www.nice.org.uk/nicemedia/pdf/Infection_control_fullguideline.pdf (accessed 29 July 2009).

NICE (2007). *NICE Clinical Guideline 54. Urinary Tract Infection in Children: Diagnosis, Treatment and Long-Term Management.* http://www.nice.org.uk/nicemedia/pdf/CG54NICEguideline.pdf (accessed 28 July 2009).

NICE (2008). *NICE Clinical Guideline 69. Respiratory Tract Infections – Antibiotic Prescribing. Prescribing of Antibiotics for Self-Limiting Respiratory Tract Infections in Adults and Children in Primary Care.* http://www.nice.org.uk/nicemedia/pdf/CG69FullGuideline.pdf (accessed 28 July 2009).

Nicolau, D.P. (2009). Containing costs and containing bugs: are they mutually exclusive? *J Manag Care Pharm 15*(2 Suppl): S12–S17.

O'Brien, F.G., Lim, T.T., Chong, F.N. et al. (2004). Diversity among community isolates of methicillin-resistant *Staphylococcus aureus* in Australia. *J Clin Microbiol 42*: 3185–3190.

Parry, C.M., Threlfall, E.J. (2008). Antimicrobial resistance in typhoidal and nontyphoidal salmonellae. *Curr Opin Infect Dis 21*(5): 531–538.

Pellowe, C.M., Pratt, R.J., Harper, P. et al. (2003). Evidence-based guidelines for preventing healthcare-associated infections in primary and community care in England. *J Hosp Infect 55* Suppl. 2: S2–S127.

Pflomm, J.M. (2002). *Strategies for minimizing antimicrobial resistance. Am J Health Syst Pharm 59* Suppl 3: S12–S15.

Plowman, R., Graves, N., Griffin, M.A. et al. (2001). The rate and cost of hospital-acquired infections occurring in patients admitted to selected specialties of a district general hospital in England and the national burden imposed. *J Hosp Infect 47*: 198–209.

Pratt, R.J., Pellowe, C.M., Wilson, J.A. et al. (2007). epic2: National evidence-based guidelines for preventing healthcare-associated infections in NHS hospitals in England. *J Hosp Infect 65S*: S1–S64.

Reeves, D. (2007). The 2005 Garrod Lecture: The changing access of patients to antibiotics – for better or worse? *J Antimicrob Chemother 59*: 333–341.

Reilly, J., Stewart, S., Allardice, G.A. et al.(2008). Results from the Scottish National HAI Prevalence Survey. *J Hosp Infect 69*(1): 62–68.

Saizy-Callaert, S., Causse, R., Furhman, C., et al. (2003). Impact of a multidisciplinary approach to the control of antibiotic prescription in a general hospital. *J Hosp Infect 53*(3): 177–182.

Schmid, D., Fretz, R., Kuo, H.W. et al. (2008). An outbreak of multidrug-resistant tuberculosis among refugees in Austria, 2005–2006. *Int J Tuberc Lung Dis 12*(10): 1190–1195.

Scottish Government (2002). *Antimicrobial Resistance Strategy and Scottish Action Plan.* http://www.scotland.gov.uk/Publications/ 2002/06/14962/7808 (accessed 29 July 2009).

Seppälä, H., Klaukka, T., Vuopio-Varkila, J. et al. (1997). The effect of changes in the consumption of macrolide antibiotics on erythromycin resistance in group A streptococci in Finland. *N Engl J Med 337*: 441–446.

Small, C.B., Bachert, C., Lund, V.J. et al. (2007). Judicious antibiotic use and intranasal corticosteroids in acute rhinosinusitis. *Am J Med 120*(4): 289–294.

Standing Medical Advisory Committee (1998) Sub-group on Antimicrobial Resistance . *The Path of Least Resistance.* London: Department of Health.

Stone, P.W., Braccia, D., Larson, E. (2005). Systematic review of economic analyses of health care-associated infections. *Am J Infect Control 33*(9): 501–509.

Sunenshine, R.H., Wright, M.O., Maragakis, L.L. et al. (2007). Multidrug-resistant Acinetobacter infection mortality rate and length of hospitalization. *Emerg Infect Dis 13*(1): 97–103.

Tapsall, J.W. (2003). Monitoring antimicrobial resistance for public health action. *Commun Dis Intell 27* Suppl: S70–S74.

Thanaviratananich, S., Laopaiboon, M., Vatanasapt, P. (2008). Once or twice daily versus three times daily amoxicillin with or without clavulanate for the treatment of acute otitis media. *Cochrane Database Syst Rev* (4): CD004975.

Tollefson, L., Karp, B.E. (2004). Human health impact from antimicrobial use in food animals. *Med Mal Infect 34*(11): 514–521.

UK Parliament (2002) Lords Hansard text for 24 January 2002 (220124–21). http://www.p ublications.parliament.uk/pa/ld200102/ldha nsrd/vo020124/text/20124–21.htm (accessed 29 July 2009).

Vouloumanou, E.K., Karageorgopoulos, D.E., Kazantzi, M.S. et al. (2009). Antibiotics versus placebo or watchful waiting for acute otitis media: a meta-analysis of randomized controlled trials. *J Antimicrob Chemother 64*(1): 16–24.

Ward, S., Lloyd Jones, M., Pandor, A. et al. (2007). A systematic review and economic evaluation of statins for the prevention of coronary events. *Health Technol Assess 11*(14): 1–160, iii-iv.

Wassenaar, T.M. (2005). Use of antimicrobial agents in veterinary medicine and implications for human health. *Crit Rev Microbiol 31*(3): 155–69.

Weinstock, D.M., Zuccotti, G. (2009). The evolution of influenza resistance and treatment. *JAMA 301*: 1066–1069.

Woodfordm, N., Ellington, M.J. (2007). The emergence of antibiotic resistance by mutation. *Clin Microbiol Infect 13*: 5–18.

Zetola, N., Francis, J.S., Nuermberger, E.L. et al. (2005). Community-acquired methicillin-resistant *Staphylococcus aureus*: an emerging threat. *Lancet Infect Dis 5*: 275–286.

Calculation skills

Alison G. Eggleton

The National Prescribing Centre (NPC) has developed competence frameworks for non-medical prescribers to assist with the maintenance of competence (NPC 2001; 2004; 2006). Each framework contains a section on prescribing safely in which one of the elements is 'checks doses and calculations to ensure accuracy and safety'. Anyone who is to check calculations performed by others must first be competent to perform such calculations. This is the most obvious element of the framework calling for competence in calculation skills. However, there are other skills called for in which competence in calculations is implicit in performing the role of a prescriber. For example, the prescriber will have access to a drug budget and must make sure that their prescribing is cost effective. The competence document makes reference to critical appraisal of literature, which will inevitably involve at least a minimal understanding of the statistical terms used by the authors. The prescriber should understand the pharmacokinetics of medicines and how changes, such as age and renal impairment, affect dosage. Again, this may require an ability to understand and utilise pharmacokinetic data.

The prescriber should know about common types of medication error and how to prevent them. The Chief Pharmaceutical Officer recognised calculation error as a key risk factor in the medication process in his 2004 report *Building a Safer NHS for Patients: Improving Medication Safety* (Smith 2004). The incorrect application of dosing equations is considered a major contributor to preventable adverse events associated with the prescribing of medicines (Lesar 1998). One major cause of adverse events is incorrect calculation of, for example, dose or rate of administration, both of which have led in the past to patient morbidity and mortality. The National Patient Safety Agency (NPSA) defines a complex calculation as any process requiring more than one step in the preparation and/or administration of a medicine to a patient (NPSA 2007), for example, when the dosage of an infusion is quoted in microgram/kg/hour. Further information on aspects of risk management with respect to calculation skills can be found in the 'Calculations' chapter in *Medication Safety: An Essential Guide* (Courtenay and Griffiths 2010).

The Nursing and Midwifery Council requires that entrants to pre-registration nursing programmes have numeracy skills sufficient to ensure proficiency in drug calculation skills relevant to professional requirements (NMC 2004) and now recommends a pass mark of 100% in the calculation assessment for independent nurse prescribers (NMC 2006). This standard should be applied to all prescribers irrespective of their particular healthcare speciality. It is therefore vital that the prescriber undertakes to develop competence in calculation skills appropriate to performance of the role.

Units of measurement

The system of measurement used in the UK is the metric system. In prescribing of medicines, probably the most commonly used units are those of mass and volume. Mass is more commonly referred to as weight and the basic metric unit is the gram (g). The basic metric unit of volume is the litre (L). Drug amounts are also commonly referred to in terms of a base unit called a mole (mol). However, it is common for multiples or fractions of these base units to be used. The prescriber must understand what these terms mean and be able to convert between dosage units accurately.

Prefixes

A prefix is a group of letters placed at the beginning of a word that change the meaning of the word. There are three prefixes commonly see in the UK metric system:

- *kilo* meaning one thousand times greater than the base unit, for example: a kilogram is 1000 grams.
- *milli* meaning one thousand times less than the base unit, for example: a milligram is 1000th of a gram.
- *micro* meaning one million times less than the base unit, for example; a microgram is 1 000 000th of a gram.

Units of volume

The base unit of volume is the litre, which is abbreviated either to L or l. The other unit of volume commonly seen is the millilitre, abbreviated to ml. One litre is equivalent to 1000 millilitres. To convert a volume in litres into a volume in millilitres, we must multiply by 1000. To convert a volume in millilitres into litres, we must divide by 1000.

For example:

Example: Convert 1.5 L into millilitres.

$$Volume\ in\ millilitres = 1.5\ L \times 1000$$
$$= 1500\ ml$$

Some people like to think of this as moving the decimal place. To multiply by 1000, you have to move the decimal place three places to the right.

$$1.5 \times 1000 = 1\ .\ 5\quad 0\quad 0$$
$$= 1500\ ml$$

Example: Convert 750 ml into litres.

$$Volume\ in\ litres = 750\ ml \div 1000$$
$$= 0.75\ L$$

Some people like to think of this as moving the decimal place. To divide by 1000, you have to move the decimal place three places to the left.

$$750 \div 1000 = \quad 7\quad 5\quad 0\ .$$
$$= \quad 0.75\ L$$

Try these examples:

1. You have a patient who needs some indigestion mixture. The usual dose is 10 ml four times a day. You decide to prescribe enough to last the patient 28 days. How much will you need to prescribe? Give your answer in litres.

   Step 1: Calculate how much the patient will take in one day.

   10 ml × 4 = 40 ml

   Step 2: Calculate how much the patient will need for 28 days.

   40 ml × 28 = 1120 ml

   Step 3: Convert the volume into litres.

   1120 ml ÷ 1000 = 1.12 L

2. You have a patient who needs to be prescribed fluids. The patient needs 35 ml fluid per kilogram body weight per day. He weighs 70 kg. How much fluid will he need in a day? Give your answer in litres.

   Step 1: Calculate how much fluid the patient will need in one day.

   35 ml × 70 = 2450 ml

   Step 2: Convert the volume into litres.

   2450 ml ÷ 1000 = 2.45 L

Units of mass

The base unit of mass, or weight as we commonly say, is the gram, which is abbreviated to g. The other units of mass commonly seen are:

- The kilogram, abbreviated to kg.
- The milligram, abbreviated to mg.
- The microgram.

Prescribers should always be very careful to write out 'microgram' **in full** and not to abbreviate it because the abbreviations that have been used (mcg or µg) have sometimes led to drug errors.

The units of mass or weight are related to each other as shown in Table 12.1.

To convert a weight in kilograms into grams, or a weight of grams into milligrams, or a weight of milligrams into micrograms, we must multiply by 1000.

Table 12.1 Units of mass

Unit	Abbreviated to	Equivalent to
1 kilogram	kg	1000 g
1 gram	g	1000 mg
1 milligram	mg	1000 microgram

For example:

Example: Convert 2.75 kg into grams.

Weight in grams = 2.75 kg × 1000
= 2750 g

Some people like to think of this as moving the decimal place. To multiply by 1000, you have to move the decimal place three places to the right.

2.75 × 1000 = 2 . 7   5   0

= 2750 g

Example: Convert 25 g into milligrams.

Weight in milligram = 25 g × 1000
= 25000 mg

Example: Convert 750 mg into micrograms.

Weight in micrograms = 750 mg × 1000
= 750000 microgram

To convert a weight in grams into kilograms, or a weight of milligrams into grams, or a weight of micrograms into milligrams, we must divide by 1000.

For example:

Example: Convert 250 microgram into milligrams.

250 ÷ 1000 = 0.25 mg

Some people like to think of this as moving the decimal place. To divide by 1000, you have to move the decimal place three places to the left.

250 ÷ 1000 =   2 5 0 .

=   0.25 mg

Example: Convert 500 mg into grams.

500 mg ÷ 1000 = 0.5 g

Example: Convert 1400 g into kilograms.

1400 ÷ 1000 = 1.4 kg

Try these examples:

1. You need to calculate the daily dose of a drug for a patient. The daily dose is 50 mg per kilogram body weight. Your patient weighs 75 kg. State your answer in grams.

   Step 1: Calculate how much drug the patient will need in one day.

   50 mg × 75 = 3750 mg

   Step 2: Convert the dose into grams.

   3750 mg ÷ 1000 = 3.75 g

2. The daily dose of immunoglobulin for a patient is 0.4 g per kilogram body weight per day. The patient weighs 70 kg. Calculate the amount needed for a five-day course. Give your answer in kilograms.

   Step 1: Calculate how much drug the patient will need in one day.

   0.4 g × 70 = 28 g

   Step 2: Calculate how much drug the patient will need for five days.

   28 g × 5 = 140 g

   Step 3: Convert into kilograms.

   140 g ÷ 1000 = 0.14 kg

3. The dose of medicine for a child is 75 microgram per kilogram body weight per day. The child weighs 15 kg. Calculate the total daily dose needed by the child in milligrams.

   Step 1: Calculate the total daily dose of the drug in micrograms.

   75 micrograms × 15 = 1125 microgram

   Step 2: Convert the total daily dose into milligrams.

   1125 microgram ÷ 1000 = 1.125 mg

4. A patient needs some cream for eczema. She needs 15 g to apply to her face, 200 g for both arms, 50 g for both hands and 400 g for her trunk. How much do you need to prescribe in total? Give your answer in kilograms.

   Step 1: Add the total amount of cream needed.

Face:	15 g
Both arms:	200 g
Both hands:	50 g
Trunk:	400 g
Total:	665 g

   Step 2: Convert the total amount into kilograms.

   665 g ÷ 1000 = 0.665 kg

Units of amount

The term used for the base unit of the amount of a drug is called a *mole*. We usually see this expressed as a mass or weight. One mole of a substance is the molecular, atomic or ionic weight of the substance expressed in grams. So, for example, one mole of sodium chloride (NaCl) would be the weight of one sodium ion (23) plus the weight of one chloride ion (35.5) expressed in grams, a total of 58.5 g. We often see the term *millimole* (meaning 1000th of a mole) when we look at a patient's biochemistry results. For example, you might see a serum potassium concentration stated as 4 mmol/L.

When we refer to a molar solution, this means that the solution contains one mole of a substance dissolved in one litre of fluid. So, for example, a molar aqueous solution of sodium chloride contains 58.5 g in one litre water. We might use this in looking at intravenous fluids. 'Normal' saline, or more correctly physiological saline, is sodium chloride solution 0.9%. This means it contains 0.9 g sodium chloride in 100 ml, or 9 g in a litre. We can work how many millimoles of sodium and chloride there are in a litre of 'normal' saline like this:

Example:
One mole of sodium chloride is 58.5 g.
A molar solution of sodium chloride contains 58.5 g in 1 L.
Therefore, a solution containing 9 g sodium chloride per litre contains:

$$9 \div 58.5 \times 1\,mole = 0.153\,mole$$

Convert this to millimoles by multiplying by 1000.

$$0.153\,mole \times 1000 = 153\,mmol$$

Therefore, one litre of a 'normal' saline contains 153 mmol sodium ions and 153 mmol chloride ions. (In practice, this is commonly rounded down and stated as 150 mmol per litre of sodium and of chloride ions.)

We will look at percentages and concentrations of solutions later (see 'Understanding concentrations').

Test yourself with practice calculations

Before you continue, test yourself with these calculations to make sure you have understood this section. Answers are given at the end of the chapter.

1. Try converting the following amounts:
   (a) How much is 1.5 kg in grams?
   (b) How much is 37.5 mg in micrograms?
   (c) How much is 650 microgram in milligrams?
   (d) How much is 1750 ml in litres?
   (e) How much is 0.95 L in millilitres?
2. You have a patient who needs the following amount of ointment for a rash all over her body. Face: 30 g, both hands: 50 g, scalp: 100 g, both arms: 200 g, both legs: 200 g, trunk 400 g, groin: 25 g. Calculate how much you should prescribe in total. Give your answer in kilograms.
3. The dose of medicine for a child is 150 microgram per kilogram body weight per day. The child weighs 25 kg. Calculate the total daily dose needed by the child in milligrams.

4. You have a patient who needs to be prescribed fluids. The patient needs 30 ml fluid per kilogram body weight per day. She weighs 65 kg. How much fluid will she need? Give your answer in litres.
5. A patient needs a mixture for indigestion. The dose needed is 20 ml four times a day. How much do you need to prescribe to last for 30 days? Give your answer in litres.

Understanding concentrations

Amount per volume

The usual method of expressing concentration of a liquid preparation that we see is an amount per unit volume. For example, you will see the following:

- micrograms per millilitre expressed as microgram/ml.
- milligrams per millilitre expressed as mg/ml.
- millimoles per litre expressed as mmol/L.
- grams per litre expressed as g/L.

We will need to use this if we are calculating the volume of a solution that we are going to administer to a patient in order to give a specified dose.

Example: If hysocine hydrobromide injection contains 400 microgram in 1 ml, how would we give a dose of 600 microgram?

Step 1: Solution contains 400 microgram in 1 ml solution.

Step 2: The volume of solution that would contain 600 microgram is:

$$\frac{600}{400} \times 1 \, ml = 1.5 \, ml$$

Example: If gentamicin injection contains 80 mg in 2 ml, how would we give a dose of 120 mg?

Step 1: Calculate the amount of gentamicin in 1 ml of solution.

Solution contains 80 mg in 2 ml.

Therefore, it contains 80 mg ÷ 2 = 40 mg in 1 ml.

Step 2: Calculate the volume of solution that contains 120 mg gentamicin.

Solution contains 40 mg in 1 ml.

Therefore, for a dose of 120 mg, we would need:

$$\frac{120}{40} \times 1 \, ml = 3 \, ml$$

Example: You need to prescribe a dose of 5 mg/kg of a drug for a child weighing 30 kg. The drug comes as a mixture that contains 100 mg of the drug in 5 ml of solution. What volume of the mixture will contain the right dose?

Step 1: Calculate the total dose of the drug.

$$5 \, mg \times 30 = 150 \, mg$$

Step 2: Calculate the volume of mixture that contains 150 mg.

Mixture contains 100 mg in 5 ml.

Therefore, the volume that contains 150 mg will be:

$$\frac{150}{100} \times 5 \, ml = 7.5 \, ml$$

Example: You need to give a dose of 2 mmol/kg of sodium to a patient weighing 20 kg. You are going to give this using sodium chloride 30% solution which contains 50 mmol sodium in 10 ml. What volume of sodium chloride 30% solution will contain the required dose?

Step 1: Calculate the total dose of the drug required.

$$2 \ mmol \times 20 = 40 \ mmol$$

Step 2: Calculate the volume of solution that contains 40 mmol.
Solution contains 50 mmol sodium in 10 ml.
Therefore, the volume that contains 40 mmol will be:

$$\frac{40}{50} \times 10 \ ml = 8 \ ml$$

Percentage concentrations

Some manufacturers express the concentration of their product as a percentage. It is important that you understand what the term percentage means so that you can work out the strength of the product. *A percentage is the amount of ingredient in 100 parts of the product.*

Percentage concentrations can be found in both solid and liquid preparations. You will see the following types of percentage expressions:

% w/v	This describes a percentage weight in volume.
	The weight will be in grams and the volume in millilitres.
	For example: sodium bicarbonate 4.2% w/v solution contains 4.2 g sodium bicarbonate in 100 ml solution.
% w/w	This describes a percentage weight in weight, most commonly of a solid. Both weights will be in grams.
	For example: betametasone 0.1% w/w cream contains 0.1 g betametasone in 100 g cream.
% v/v	This describes a percentage volume in volume of a liquid. Both volumes will be in millilitres.
	For example: liquid paraffin oral emulsion 50% v/v contains 50 ml liquid paraffin in 100 ml emulsion.

Example: How much lidocaine is contained in 5 ml of lidocaine 2% injection?
Step 1: Work out what the percentage strength means in gram per 100 ml.
Lidocaine 2% injection contains 2 g lidocaine in 100 ml solution.
Step 2: Convert the strength of solution to milligrams in 100 ml.

$$2 \ g \ in \ 100 \ ml = 2 \times 1000 \ mg \ in \ 100 \ ml$$
$$= 2000 \ mg \ in \ 100 \ ml$$

Step 3: Calculate how much lidocaine there is in 5 ml of the solution.

$$\frac{5}{100} \times 2000 = 100 \ mg \ in \ 5 \ ml$$

Example: How much bupivacaine is contained in 10 ml of bupivacaine 0.5% injection?
Step 1: Work out what the percentage strength means in gram per 100 ml.

Bupivacaine 0.5% injection contains 0.5 g bupivacaine in 100 ml solution.

Step 2: Convert the strength of solution to milligrams in 100 ml.

0.5 g in 100 ml = 0.5 × 1000 mg in 100 ml

= 500 mg in 100 ml

Step 3: Calculate how much bupivacaine there is in 10 ml of the solution.

$$\frac{10}{100} \times 500 = 50 \text{ mg in 10 ml}$$

Concentrations expressed in ratios or parts

A ratio concentration is often used to describe the concentration of very dilute solutions. It expresses the number of grams of a drug that are dissolved or dispersed in a given number of parts of a solution in millilitres. For example, adrenaline solution 1 in 1000 contains 1 g adrenaline in 1000 ml of solution. Because these solutions tend to be very dilute and yet very potent, we must be particularly careful with these calculations.

Example: How much adrenaline is contained in 1 ml of adrenaline 1 in 1000 solution?

Step 1: Work out what the ratio strength means.

Adrenaline 1 in 1000 = 1 g in 1000 ml

Step 2: Convert the strength of solution to milligrams.

1 g in 1000 ml = 1 × 1000 mg in 1000 ml

= 1000 mg in 1000 ml

Step 3: Calculate how much adrenaline there is in 1 ml of the solution.

$$\frac{1}{1000} \times 1000 = 1 \text{ mg in 1 ml}$$

Example: How much adrenaline is contained in 10 ml of adrenaline 1 in 10 000 dilute solution?

Step 1: Work out what the ratio strength means.

Adrenaline 1 in 10 000 = 1 g in 10 000 ml

Step 2: Convert the strength of solution to milligrams.

1 g in 10 000 ml = 1 × 1000 mg in 10 000 ml

= 1000 mg in 10 000 ml

Step 3: calculate how much adrenaline there is in 10 ml of the solution.

$$\frac{10}{10000} \times 1000 = 1 \text{ mg in 10 ml}$$

Test yourself with practice calculations

Before you continue, test yourself with these calculations to make sure you have understood this section. Answers are given at the end of the chapter.

6. How much potassium permanganate is contained in 100 ml of potassium permanganate 1 in 10 000 solution?
7. How much hydrogen peroxide is contained in 250 ml of hydrogen peroxide 6% solution?
8. You have levomepromazine injection 25 mg in 1 ml. You want to put a dose of 6.25 mg into a syringe driver. What volume of levomepromazine injection do you need?
9. You want to give a dose of 25 mg per kilogram of a drug to a child weighing 18 kg. The solution you have contains 200 mg in 5 ml. What volume of the solution will contain the right dose?
10. You want to give a bolus dose of 100 mg lidocaine to a patient to control ventricular arrhythmia. The injection solution you have is lidocaine injection 2%. What volume of the injection do you need to give this dose?

Calculating the dose

The 'dose' of a drug is the amount of drug given to the patient to achieve a therapeutic outcome. The calculated dose may be given as a total daily dose in a single administration (such as digoxin 125 microgram daily) or it may be necessary to divide the dose into smaller amounts given on more than one occasion during the day (such as diclofenac 50 mg three times a day). There are certain patient groups, like children for example, where the need for dose calculation is common. A prescriber must take care to understand clearly statements about dosage and to calculate doses accurately. The dosage statement may, for example, give the amount to be given *per dose* or the amount to be given *in total per day*, which then needs to be divided according to the recommended frequency of administration. The prescriber may also need to round calculated doses up or down in order to match with availability of a drug formulation. For example, for dissolution of gallstones, the dose of ursodeoxycholic acid in the BNF is 8–12 mg/kg daily as a single dose at bedtime or in two divided doses (BNF 2008). For a patient weighing 60 kg, the total daily dose would be 480–720 mg. The product is available as tablets of 150 mg or capsules of 250 mg. Therefore, in order to keep within the recommended dosage range, the prescribed dose could be, say, 500 mg daily or 250 mg twice daily.

Dosage calculations can be based on (Bonner et al. 2001):

- A given amount of drug per kilogram body weight of the patient.
- A given amount of drug based on a patient's body surface area.
- A given rate of drug administration per unit time (see 'Calculating the rate of drug administration per unit time' below).

Dosage calculations can sometimes be based on a patient's ideal body weight rather than actual body weight. The following equations can be used to calculate the ideal body weight.

Male: Ideal body weight $= (0.9 \times \text{height in centimetres}) - 88 \text{ kg}$

Female: Ideal body weight $= (0.9 \times \text{height in centimetres}) - 92 \text{ kg}$

Calculating a dose based on a patient's body weight

Try these examples:

Example: Calculate the dose of co-amoxiclav suspension 250/62 for a child aged 7 years weighing 23 kg.

(Note: when selecting doses for children, the *BNF for Children* should normally be used. These examples are quoted from the dosage statements in the standard BNF for the purposes of practising the calculation technique only.)

Step 1: Check the recommended dose in the BNF. The stated dose of co-amoxiclav 250/62 for a child aged 6–12 years is 0.4 ml/kg body weight daily given in three divided doses, increased to 0.8 ml/kg body weight in severe infections. We are going to use 0.4 ml/kg/day.

Step 2: Calculate the total daily dose.

$$\text{Daily dose at 0.4 ml/kg} = \text{Patient's weight (kg)} \times \text{Daily dose (ml/kg)}$$
$$= 23 \text{ kg} \times 0.4 \text{ ml/kg per day}$$
$$= 9.2 \text{ ml per day}$$

Step 3: Calculate the dose to be given three times a day.

$$= 9.2 \text{ ml} \div 3$$
$$= 3.07 \text{ ml}$$

Step 4: Convert the dose into a practical dosage for administration to the patient.

A practical dose to prescribe would be 3 ml three times a day.

Example: Calculate the dose of salbutamol oral solution for a child aged 6 months weighing 7.8 kg. The dose of salbutamol stated in the BNF for a child aged 6 months is 100 microgram/kg body weight four times a day (unlicensed use).

Step 1: Calculate the amount per dose.

$$\text{Amount per dose at 100 microgram/kg} = \text{Patient's weight (kg)} \times \text{Amount per dose}$$
$$\text{(microgram/kg)}$$
$$= 7.8 \text{ kg} \times 100 \text{ microgram/kg}$$
$$= 780 \text{ microgram per dose}$$

Step 2: Calculate the volume of salbutamol oral solution that contains 780 microgram.

Salbutamol oral solution contains 2 mg salbutamol in 5 ml. To make sure we don't mix up the units we should convert this to a strength stated as micrograms in 5 ml.

$$2 \text{ mg in 5 ml} = (2 \times 1000 \text{ microgram}) \text{ in 5 ml}$$
$$= 2000 \text{ microgram in 5 ml}$$

Therefore, the amount of the oral solution that contains a dose of 780 microgram would be:

$$\frac{780}{2000} \times 5 \text{ ml} = 1.95 \text{ ml}$$

Step 3: convert this dose into a practical dose for administration to the patient.

Oral syringes for children are available in various sizes. It would probably be best to round this dose up to 2 ml. Therefore the dose to prescribe would be 2 ml four times a day of salbutamol 2 mg in 5 ml oral solution.

Example: Calculate the dose of gentamicin for an adult male patient to treat septicaemia. The dose should be based on ideal body weight. The patient weighs 85 kg and is 180 cm tall.

(Note: many hospitals now use a once-daily gentamicin dosing regime rather than this multiple dosing regime. This example is quoted from the dosage statement in the standard

BNF for the purposes of practising the calculation technique only. Prescribers should refer to their local gentamicin prescribing guidelines.)

Step 1: Check the recommended dose in the BNF. The stated adult dose of gentamicin is 3–5 mg/kg body weight daily given in divided doses every eight hours. We are going to use 5 mg/kg/day to treat septicaemia.

Step 2: Calculate the patient's ideal body weight.

Male: Ideal body weight (IBW) $= (0.9 \times \text{height in centimetres}) - 88 \text{ kg}$

$$= (0.9 \times 180) - 88 \text{ kg}$$

$$= 74 \text{ kg}$$

Step 3: Calculate the total daily dose.

Daily dose at 5 mg/kg $= \text{Patient's IBW (kg)} \times \text{Daily dose (mg/kg)}$

$$= 74 \text{ kg} \times 5 \text{ mg/kg per day}$$

$$= 370 \text{ mg per day}$$

Step 4: Calculate the dose to be given every eight hours:

$$= 370 \text{ mg} \div 3$$

$$= 123.3 \text{ mg per dose}$$

Step 5: Convert the dose into a practical dosage for administration to the patient. Gentamicin injection is available in a strength of 40 mg in 1 ml.

Therefore a practical dose to prescribe would be 120 mg every eight hours (three times a day).

Step 6: Calculate the volume of gentamicin injection that contains 120 mg.

If gentamicin injection contains 40 mg in 1 ml, a dose of 120 mg would be equivalent to:

$$\frac{120}{40} \times 1 \text{ ml} = 3 \text{ ml}$$

The dose of gentamicin based on ideal body weight would therefore be 120 mg (3 ml) every eight hours of gentamicin 40 mg in 1 ml injection.

Calculating the dose based on a patient's body surface area

Some dosage calculations are based on the patient's body surface area (BSA) as opposed to body weight. BSA calculations were originally introduced to work out safe starting doses in the early stages of trials of drugs in humans which had previously only been tested in animals. It has become routine practice for dosing of many anti-cancer drugs, although response (or toxicity) is not always closely related to BSA. Calculations used in adult oncology were originally constructed from a study by DuBois and DuBois (1916). This study utilised only nine patients and its accuracy has been disputed (DuBois and DuBois 1916; Wang et al. 1992). However, because the method is still widely used, prescribers involved in oncology will need to be able to calculate the dosage of drugs using this method.

In general, BSA is estimated using a nomogram. Prescribers must be careful to select the correct nomogram because different ones are available for adults and children. Prescribing in oncology is a specialised and high-risk field of practice. These calculation examples are merely included to raise awareness of this method of calculating doses. *Anyone anticipating working in the field of oncology must ensure that further specialist training in dosage calculation is undertaken.*

Example: Calculate the dose of cyclophosphamide using the low-dose intravenous regimen for an adult patient with a BSA estimated at 2.2 m^2.

Step 1: Check the recommended dose in the manufacturer's Summary of Product Characteristics for cyclophosphamide (EMC 2007). This is stated as follows:

Low dose: 80–240 mg/m^2 as a single dose weekly intravenously.

Say we chose 80 mg/m^2.

Step 2: Calculate the dose for a patient with a BSA of 2.2 m^2.

$$\text{Weekly dose} = 80 \text{ mg/m}^2 \times 2.2 \text{ m}^2$$
$$= 176 \text{ mg}$$

In general, doses of cytotoxic drugs are not rounded up or down but are prepared individually for the patient, although dose banding is used in some organisations, partly for the convenience of batch production and partly as a risk reduction strategy (MacLean et al. 2003). In dose banding, a selection of pre-prepared syringes is used to make up the dose to within 5% of the patient's calculated dose. Cyclophosphamide is one of the drugs described as being suitable for dose banding.

Example: Calculate the *intravenous* dose of vincristine for a child with a BSA estimated at 0.6 m^2. The suggested dose of vincristine is 1.4 to 2 mg/m^2 once a week up to a maximum of 2 mg once-weekly (EMC 2009). For children weighing 10 kg or less the starting dose should be 0.05 mg/kg once a week. The dose we are going to use in our calculation is 2 mg/kg.

(Note: The National Patient Safety Agency requires that a register is maintained of all persons involved in the prescribing, dispensing, delivery and administration of vinca alkaloids (DoH 2001; 2003; NPSA 2008). Vincristine is a high-risk drug. You must not prescribe vincristine or any other vinca alkaloid unless you are specifically authorised and trained to do so and your name appears on the risk register maintained within your employing organisation. This example is included for the purposes of calculation practice only.)

Step 1: Calculate the dose for a child with a BSA of 0.6 m^2.

$$\text{Weekly IV dose} = 2 \text{ mg/m}^2 \times 0.6 \text{ m}^2$$
$$= 1.2 \text{ mg}$$

Test yourself with practice calculations

Before you continue, test yourself with these calculations to make sure you have understood this section. Answers are given at the end of the chapter.

11. What is the ideal body weight of the following patients?
    a. A man who is 185 cm tall?
    b. A woman who is 150 cm tall?
12. What is the dose of co-amoxiclav suspension 125/35 for a child aged 3 years weighing 16 kg? The dose in the standard BNF is 0.8 ml/kg daily given in three divided doses, increased to 1.6 ml/kg daily in three divided doses for severe infections. Use 0.8 ml/kg daily in your calculation.
13. Calculate the dose of tobramycin for an adult female to treat a severe infection to be given by slow intravenous bolus injection. The dose recommended in the BNF is 3 mg/kg daily in divided doses every eight hours. The dose must be based on ideal body weight. The patient is 165 cm tall.

14. Calculate the dose of cyclophosphamide using the low-dose intravenous regimen for an adult patient with a BSA estimated at 1.95 m². The selected dose is 120 mg/m² once a week.

Calculating the rate of drug administration per unit time

Calculating the rate of administration of an infusion to be given using a volumetric infusion device set in drops per minute

An *adult* volumetric giving set administers 1 ml for every 20 drops of solution.

(Note: care is needed. This value is different for blood giving sets and for paediatric giving sets. Always check the number of drops per ml for the giving set you are using.)

Say you wanted to administer 1 L of glucose 5% infusion over eight hours.

Step 1: Convert the volume of solution into millilitres.

1 L over 8 hours = 1000 ml over 8 hours

Step 2: Calculate the volume of solution to be given per hour.

$$1000 \text{ ml over 8 hours} = \frac{1000 \text{ ml}}{8} = 125 \text{ ml per hour}$$

Step 3: Calculate the volume of solution to be given per minute.

$$125 \text{ ml over 1 hour} = \frac{125}{60} = 2.08 \text{ ml per minute}$$

This could be rounded down to 2 ml per minute as this method of administration is not accurate to two decimal places.

Step 4: Calculate the number of drops equivalent to this volume.

Using our chosen giving set, we must administer 20 drops to give 1 ml solution.

Therefore 2 ml = 40 drops.

Therefore the drip controller should be set so that it administers 40 drops in one minute in order to administer 1 L of fluid over eight hours.

Calculating the rate of administration of an infusion to be given using a high-risk infusion device set in millilitres per hour

Administration of drugs by the intravenous route is a high-risk procedure. Hospital pharmacists generally try to help make this procedure safer by producing monographs for intravenous administration. Often, for high-risk drugs, such as dopamine, a standard table of administration according to rate of administration and patient's weight will be available. However, health professionals should be aware of how such tables are calculated.

Before administering a drug intravenously, you should check:

- That the situation of the patient matches the monograph. For example, some drugs can only be given in critical care areas with appropriate close monitoring of the patient.

- That the drug can be given through the available intravenous line. For example, some drugs can be given only via a central line.
- That the drug can be given through the available intravenous line in the concentration prescribed. For example, the concentration of some drug solutions varies according to whether a central or peripheral line is used.
- That the patient details correspond with the types of patient mentioned in the monograph. For example, there will be different monographs for adults, children and neonates.
- The dose to be administered. The monograph will normally include a statement of the correct dose to be administered according to the indication.
- The diluent. Some drugs can only be diluted in certain diluents.

Example: Calculate the rate of administration in millilitres per hour of dopamine infusion for a patient weighing 60 kg. You have been asked to give dopamine to go through a peripheral line at a rate of 3 microgram/kg/minute diluted in normal saline. The patient is on a general medical ward. The recommended dilution of the infusion for peripheral administration is 800 mg dopamine in 500 ml normal saline.

Step 1: Calculate the dose in microgram/min for a 60 kg patient.

Dopamine is to be given at a rate of 3 microgram/kg/min. The patient weighs 60 kg.

$$3 \text{ microgram} \times 60 \text{ kg} = 180 \text{ microgram per minute}$$

Step 2: Calculate the dose in microgram/hour for a 60 kg patient.

$$180 \text{ microgram/min} \times 60 \text{mins} = 10\,800 \text{ microgram per hour}$$

Step 3: Convert the dose into milligram/hour.

$$1 \text{ mg} = 1000 \text{ microgram}$$

$$\text{Therefore } 10\,800 \text{ microgram} = 10.8 \text{ mg per hour}$$

Step 4: Check the recommended dilution of the solution for the infusion method selected and convert the calculated dose into a practical dose for administration.

The recommended dilution of the infusion for peripheral administration is 800 mg dopamine in 500 ml normal saline. What would be the rate of administration in millilitres per hour to achieve a rate of 10.8 mg per hour?

If a solution contains 800 mg in 500 ml, how much does it contain in 1 ml?

$$\frac{1 \text{ ml}}{500 \text{ ml}} \times 800 \text{ mg} = 1.6 \text{ mg in 1 ml}$$

Therefore, how much of the solution would contain 10.8 mg?

$$\frac{10.8 \text{ mg}}{1.6 \text{ mg}} \times 1 \text{ ml} = 6.75 \text{ ml per hour}$$

Calculating a dose for a patient on a milligram per kilogram basis

Example: Calculate the dose of aminophylline to treat an adult with an acute severe asthma attack. Assume that the patient has not previously been treated with theophylline or aminophylline.

The patient weighs 85 kg. You need to give a loading dose of 5 mg per kg given over 20 minutes then a maintenance dose of 500 mcg/kg/hour. The solution of aminophylline is made up as 500 mg in 500 ml.

Step 1: Calculate the loading dose.

$$5 \text{ mg per kg} \times 85\text{kg} = 425 \text{ mg over 20 mins in either normal saline}$$
$$\text{or glucose 5\% infusion.}$$

Step 2: Calculate the maintenance dose.

$$500 \text{ mcg/kg/hr in a patient weighing 85 kg} = 500 \times 85 \text{ mcg/hr}$$
$$= 42\,500 \text{ mcg/hr}$$

Step 3: Convert to milligram per hour.

$$42\,500 \text{ mcg/hr} = (42\,500 \div 1000) \text{ mg/hr}$$
$$= 42.5 \text{ mg/hr}$$

Step 4: Calculate the rate of administration.
The solution contains 500 mg in 500 ml, or 1 mg in 1 ml.
Therefore the maintenance infusion should be set at 42.5 ml/hr.

Test yourself with practice calculations

15. A patient requires 1 L of normal saline to be given over 12 hours. What is the correct rate for the drip controller in drops per minute assuming the giving set delivers 20 drops for 1 ml of solution?
16. A patient requires 500 ml glucose 5% to be given over three hours. What is the correct rate for the drip controller in drops per minute assuming the giving set delivers 20 drops for 1 ml of solution?
17. Calculate the rate of administration in millilitres per hour of dobutamine infusion to be administered at a rate of 2.5 microgram/kg/minute to a patient weighing 75 kg. The solution should be made up (according to the IV monograph for critical care areas) as dobutamine 250 mg in 500 ml sodium chloride 0.9% infusion.
18. Calculate the rate of administration in millilitres per hour of dopamine infusion to be administered at a rate of 2 microgram/kg/minute to a patient weighing 65 kg. The solution should be made up (according to the IV monograph) as dopamine 800mg (4 ampoules) in 500 ml fluid.
19. Calculate the dose of aminophylline infusion to treat an adult with an acute severe asthma attack. Assume that the patient has not previously been treated with theophylline or aminophylline. The patient weighs 65 kg. You need to prescribe a loading dose of 5 mg per kg given over 20 minutes then a maintenance dose of 500 mcg/kg/hour. The solution of aminophylline is made up as 500 mg in 500 ml.
20. Calculate the dose of ciclosporin to treat a patient with severe active rheumatoid arthritis. The oral dose is 2.5 mg/kg daily in two divided doses. The patient weighs 65 kg. The capsules are available in 25 mg, 50 mg and 100 mg strengths only.

Calculating unit costs of drugs

One of the competencies for supplementary and independent prescribers is to prescribe in a cost-effective way. There is a science which looks at cost-effectiveness and clinical effectiveness of drugs called pharmacoeconomics. We are not trying to look at this topic in the amount of detail needed for a full pharmacoeconomic analysis. Here, we will be looking at a way of calculating the cost of treatment courses of drugs so that a simple cost comparison may be made.

Example:

a. **How to work out the cost of a medicine per day**

What information do you need?

Cost per pack.

Number of dose units in the pack.

Number of dose units used per day.

Example:

Cimetidine Tablets 400 mg

Cost per pack = £1.55 (BNF no 56 price)

Number of tablets in a pack = 60

Daily dose: 2 tablets per day

You may find it easier to convert the cost of the pack into pence here so that you know the answer will be in pence.

Calculate the cost per tablet:

60 tablets = £1.55 = 155 pence

$$1 \text{ tablet} = \frac{155}{60} = 2.58 \text{ pence (rounded up to 3 pence)}$$

Calculate the cost per day:

3 pence per tablet × 2 tablets per day = 6 pence per day

b. **How to work out the cost per treatment course**

What information do you need?

Cost per day.

Number of weeks or days in the course.

Example:

Cimetidine Tablets 400 mg

Cost per day = 6 pence

Number of weeks in the course = 8 weeks

Therefore number of days in the course = 8 × 7 = 56 days

Calculate the cost per course:

6 pence per day × 56 days = 336 pence = £3.36

In the real situation, if you wanted to compare cimetidine with other histamine H_2 antagonists, you would also need to consider how long the treatment course was for each drug, what percentage of patients were cured by the standard treatment course, what the comparative relapse rates were, etc. However, this method would enable you to compare different treatment regimes in terms of drug cost alone.

Test yourself with practice calculations

21. Calculate the comparative *monthly* treatment costs of the following non-steroidal anti-inflammatory (NSAID) drugs.

Drug	Pack size	Cost per pack	Treatment course	Daily dose
Ibuprofen tabs 400 mg	84	£2.24	28 days	400 mg TDS
Diclofenac tabs 50 mg	84	£1.79	28 days	50 mg TDS
Naproxen tabs 500 mg	28	£1.65	28 days	500 mg BD

22. Calculate the monthly treatment costs of the following antacids assuming they are taken regularly in the dose listed in the table, in each case the upper end of the recommended dosage range.

Drug	Pack size	Cost per pack	Treatment course	Daily dose
Gastrocote® liquid	500 ml	£2.67	28 days	15 ml QDS
Gaviscon Advance® liquid	250 ml	£2.70	28 days	20 ml QDS
Peptac suspension	500 ml	£2.16	28 days	10 ml QDS

Simple pharmacokinetic calculations

Pharmacokinetics is a topic included within the core curriculum for independent and supplementary prescribing. Pharmacokinetic calculations can be very complex and you may need a specialist practitioner, such as a clinical pharmacist, to help you with them. However, some simple calculations can help you when you are counselling your patients on their medication. They can also help when you are converting between routes of administration of a drug.

Half-life

The half-life of a drug is the time taken for the plasma concentration to reduce by half. It is relatively constant for a given drug, assuming no change in the patient's liver or renal function, although in some cases there may be wide inter-patient variation. So why is half-life important?

When a patient starts taking a drug and continues to take it regularly at the prescribed intervals, the blood level of the drug gradually increases until it becomes constant. This constant blood level is called the *'steady state plasma concentration'*. For a drug with a simple pharmacokinetic profile, although it may begin to take effect after the first dose, it will generally not reach its full effect until steady state plasma concentration is reached. This will be after four to five times the half-life of a drug. Table 12.2 shows you why this is the case.

The patient is given a dose at time zero and it will achieve a certain blood level. After one half-life, the blood level will have fallen to half its original value, say 10 mg/L, as the drug is excreted. After a second half-life it will fall by half again to 5 mg/L. After a third half-life it will

Table 12.2 Plasma concentration after repeated oral dosing of a drug (where the dose interval is the same as the half-life)

Number of half-lives	Number of doses	Plasma concentration remaining from each dose (mg/L)						Total plasma concentration
1	1	10.00						10.00
2	2	5.00	10.00					15.00
3	3	2.50	5.00	10.00				17.50
4	4	1.25	2.50	5.00	10.00			18.75
5	5	0.625	1.25	2.50	5.00	10.00		19.38
6	6	0.3125	0.625	1.25	2.50	5.00	10.00	19.69

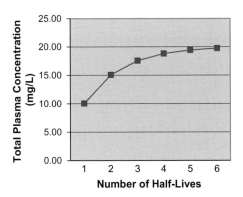

Figure 12.1 Increasing total plasma concentration with number of half-lives at the beginning of dosing

fall by half again to 2.5 mg/L and so on. But say we give more doses. Each dose will achieve the original blood level and start falling off as it is excreted. Each time a dose is given, a portion of that dose will be retained at each half-life. All of these portions together add up to make the total blood level (or total plasma concentration). We can see from Figure 12.1 that the plasma concentration starts to flatten out at around five half-lives and this is the steady state plasma concentration.

The reverse is true when the patient stops taking a drug. The initial blood level will be the steady state plasma concentration. When the patient stops taking the drug, the blood level will fall to half of its original concentration at each half-life. Therefore, as we can see from Table 12.3, it will take about four to five times the half-life of a drug to eliminate the drug from the body.

Understanding the term half-life of a drug is important for various reasons:

Time taken for medication to reach maximum effect. Consider ibuprofen with its half-life of about two hours (Setter and Baker 2002). If a patient started taking ibuprofen for pain relief, there would be some effect from the first dose when it reached the initial peak plasma concentration after about an hour. However, in order to obtain maximum therapeutic effect, the patient would need to continue taking the drug regularly according to the recommended dosing schedule. Steady state plasma concentration, and thus maximum pain relief, would be reached after about eight to ten hours (four to five times the half life of two hours). Patient confidence in the prescriber is likely to be increased if this type of information can be given.

Table 12.3 Plasma concentration at the end of dosing of a drug

Number of half-lives	Total plasma concentration (mg/L)
0	20.00
1	10.00
2	5.00
3	2.50
4	1.25
5	0.625

Example: Naproxen is a non-steroidal anti-inflammatory drug with a half-life of about 14 hours (Setter and Baker 2002). If you prescribed this drug and the patient took it regularly according to the recommended dosing schedule, how long would it take to reach steady state plasma concentration?

Step 1: Shortest time to steady state plasma concentration:

$= 4 \times 14$ hours

$= 56$ hours

Step 2: Longest time to steady state plasma concentration:

$= 5 \times 14$ hours

$= 70$ hours

Time for the effect of medication to wear off. Some drugs have a very long half-life. If a patient was getting side effects and the decision was taken to discontinue the drug, it would take four to five half-lives for the drug to be eliminated and for its effect to wear off completely. For example, if a patient was taking digoxin, with a half-life of about 40 hours (Bauman 2002) (assuming normal renal function), it would take over a week to eliminate digoxin from the bloodstream. Any toxic effects would wear off sometime during that week as the blood level fell.

Example: A patient was taking digoxin but was getting toxic effects including nausea and diarrhoea. A blood level was reported as 2.8 nanogram/ml. If the patient stopped taking digoxin, how long would it take for the blood level to fall to 0.35 nanogram/ml? Assume that the half-life of digoxin in this patient is 40 hours.

Step 1: After one half-life (40 hours), the digoxin level will have reduced by half.

2.8 nanogram/ml ÷ 2 = 1.4 nanogram/ml

Step 2: After a second half-life (40 hours), the digoxin level will have reduced by half again.

1.4 nanogram/ml ÷ 2 = 0.7 nanogram/ml

Step 3: After a third half-life (40 hours), the digoxin level will have reduced by half again.

0.7 nanogram/ml ÷ 2 = 0.35 nanogram/ml

Step 4: Therefore the digoxin level will fall to 0.35 nanogram/ml after 3 x half-life

half-life = 3×40 hours = 120 hours.

Change of half-life depending on the patient. The half-life of a drug is relatively constant in a given patient group but it can vary between different patient groups. For example, because digoxin is renally excreted, its half-life is extended in patients with poor renal function, up to four to five days (Bauman 2002). Some drugs have a different half-life in children because of their different body composition and systems for eliminating drugs. Gentamicin, for example, has a half-life of about two hours in a normal adult, but about three hours in an older infant, or about 50–70 hours in an adult patient with anuria (Mercier 2002a).

This information about half-life is something of a generalisation because:

- The clinical effect of some drugs is not directly related to the plasma concentration. Tricyclic antidepressants used to treat depression and disease-modifying drugs used to treat rheumatoid arthritis are two examples of drugs known to take a few weeks to take effect.

- Some drugs are metabolised to produce active metabolites. These metabolites will have their own half-lives. The effect of the drug may be related to the half-life of the metabolite(s), not just the drug itself. For example, the serum level of chlorphenamine does not correlate with its histamine antagonist activity because of an active metabolite (Marshik 2002).

- Genetic differences between patients can mean that there is wide inter-patient variation in steady state plasma levels. For example, there can be a 30-fold variation in steady state plasma level between patients taking the same dose of heterocyclic antidepressants (Stimmel 2002).

Bioavailability

Bioavailability of a drug is the fraction of the dose administered that reaches the systemic circulation. It estimates the *extent* but not the rate of absorption. For an intravenous injection, the bioavailability is 100% because all of the dose is put directly into the systemic circulation. If a drug is given by another route of administration, then less than 100% of the drug may reach the bloodstream. This may be due to a variety of causes, such as extensive metabolism of the drug in the liver, the relative lipid and water solubility of the drug molecule that determines whether it will cross cell membranes, breakdown of the drug in the gastrointestinal tract and many other factors. It is not possible to administer some drugs orally because the amount of drug reaching the systemic circulation via this route is negligible.

Once a drug has been marketed, the manufacturer will have designed a dosage form that will allow sufficient drug into the bloodstream to have the required clinical effect. However, it is important to know about relative bioavailability of different dosage forms of the same drug to determine if a dosage change is required when the route of administration is changed. A good example of this would be benzylpenicillin (penicillin G). When given intravenously, 100% of the injection reaches the bloodstream. However, when given orally only 15–30% of the drug is absorbed because the drug is broken down by acid in the stomach. It is common to give penicillin V if the oral route is required because it has more complete (60%) and more reliable oral absorption (Mercier 2002b).

A knowledge of bioavailability is important if changing from one route of administration to another. Here are some examples:

- Carbamazepine can be given by mouth to treat, among other things, epilepsy. If the patient is unable to take medication by the oral route, suppositories are available but a dose of 100 mg orally is equivalent to a dose of 125 mg rectally (BNF 2008). An additional problem is that absorption from carbamazepine suppositories is saturable and the maximum to be given per dose is 250 mg. Therefore a change of dosage frequency may also be needed.

Example: A patient has been stabilised on an oral dose of carbamazepine of 300 mg twice a day. What is the equivalent dose in suppositories?

Step 1: Total daily dose of carbamazepine = 300 mg × 2 = 600 mg.

Step 2: Convert 600 mg orally to the equivalent in suppositories.

$$100 \text{ mg orally} = 125 \text{ mg rectally}$$

$$\text{Therefore, } 600 \text{ mg orally} = (6 \times 125 \text{ mg}) \text{ rectally}$$

$$= 750 \text{ mg}$$

Step 3: No more than 250 mg can be given at a time by the rectal route. Therefore a rectal dose of 750 mg must be given as 250 mg three times a day.

- Sodium fucidate tablets are given by mouth to treat staphylococcal infections. The usual adult dose of the tablets is 500 mg three times a day. If the patient requires a liquid preparation, the suspension contains fusidic acid, which is less completely absorbed. The usual adult dose of the suspension is 750 mg three times a day (BNF 2008).
- Phenytoin sodium, another anti-epileptic drug, is given by mouth in capsule form commonly in a dose of 150–300 mg daily. If the patient requires a liquid preparation, the suspension contains phenytoin base. The conversion recommended in the BNF is that phenytoin sodium 100 mg (capsule) is equivalent therapeutically to phenytoin 90 mg (suspension or liquid) (BNF 2008).

Example: A patient has been stabilised on an oral dose of phenytoin sodium capsules of 300 mg daily. What is the equivalent dose of phenytoin liquid?

Step 1: Phenytoin sodium capsule 100 mg = phenytoin liquid 90 mg.

Step 2: Phenytoin sodium capsule (3 × 100 mg).

$$= \text{phenytoin liquid } (3 \times 90 \text{ mg})$$

$$= \text{phenytoin liquid } 270 \text{ mg}$$

Step 3: Phenytoin liquid contains 30 mg phenytoin in 5 ml. Therefore what volume contains 270 mg?

$$\frac{270 \text{ mg}}{30 \text{ mg}} \times 5 \text{ ml} = 45 \text{ ml}$$

Test yourself with practice calculations

Before you continue, test yourself with these calculations to make sure you have understood this section. Answers are given at the end of the chapter.

23. What is the time to steady state plasma concentration of the following drugs? Assume that steady state is reached after five half-lives and that the drug is taken regularly by the patient.

Drug	Half-life (Setter and Baker 2002)
Paracetamol	2 hours
Indomethacin	2.4 hours
Meloxicam	20 hours
Piroxicam	48 hours

24. A patient has been taking theophylline and has a toxic plasma level of 28 mg/L. The half-life of theophylline in this patient is estimated as eight hours. How long would it take for the plasma concentration to fall within reference range for theophylline (10–15 mg/L)?

25. You have an epileptic patient who has been taking phenytoin sodium capsules 350 mg daily for several weeks and is well controlled. However, she has had a stroke and can no longer swallow the capsules. What is the equivalent dose of phenytoin suspension?

26. You have an epileptic patient who has been taking carbamazepine 400 mg twice daily for several weeks and is well controlled. However, she is nil by mouth at the moment. What is the equivalent dose in suppositories?

Palliative care

Syringe drivers

In palliative care, patients often receive drugs via a syringe driver. The legislation surrounding prescribing of controlled drugs is constantly changing with respect to independent nurse prescribing, patient group directions and supplementary prescribing. Prescribers must make sure they are aware of the current legislation using an up-to-date source such as the Department of Health website.

Caution: when drugs are combined in a syringe driver, this is off-licence prescribing. The prescriber assumes liability for the final product. Compatibility of the resulting solution must ALWAYS be checked using a specialist medicines information source such as a palliative care handbook. Compatibility will depend on:

- *The drug combination used.*
- *The diluent used to make up the solution.*
- *The final concentration of each ingredient in the solution.*

Prescribers should be aware of how to calculate the ingredients in a syringe driver in the event that they make up the device content for administration to the patient and also so that appropriate quantities of injection solutions can be prescribed.

We have already looked at how to calculate the volume of injection containing a given dose of medication. Here is a reminder:

Example: If metoclopramide injection contains 10 mg in 1 ml, what volume contains 15 mg?

$$\frac{15}{10} \times 1 = 1.5 \, \text{ml}$$

Example: If hyoscine hydrobromide injection contains 400 microgram in 1 ml, what volume contains 300 microgram?

$$\frac{300}{400} \times 1 = 0.75 \text{ ml}$$

In order to calculate the content of a syringe driver, we must calculate the volume of each injection solution to be added. We must also know the final volume of the syringe driver we are intending to make up so that we can work out how much diluent we need.

Example: If we wanted to make up a syringe driver to contain diamorphine 10 mg (reconstituted with 1 ml water for injection) and cyclizine 50 mg (1 ml) and the final volume of the syringe driver was 10 ml, the amount of water for injection that would be required is (10 ml – 1 ml – 1 ml) = 8 ml. Therefore the prescriber would need to ensure the patient had a supply of 10 ml vials of water for injection to be able to make up the final volume.

Calculation of breakthrough analgesia doses

If morphine is being given in the form of slow-release tablets, patients are usually prescribed a dose of non-slow-release morphine to take when needed for breakthrough pain. Non-slow-release morphine acts for about four hours and is therefore usually given up to six times a day. This is used to provide a formula for calculating how big the breakthrough dose should be:

$$\textbf{Breakthrough dose} = \frac{(\textbf{total daily dose of slow - release morphine})}{6}$$

Example: If a patient is taking morphine sulphate slow-release tablets 120 mg twice a day, what should the breakthrough dose of non-slow-release morphine be?

Step 1: Total daily dose of slow-release morphine = 120 mg × 2 = 240 mg.
Step 2: Breakthrough dose of non-slow-release morphine is:

$$\frac{240 \text{ mg}}{6} = 40 \text{ mg}$$

A dose of 40 mg non-slow-release morphine should be prescribed to be taken when required for breakthrough pain.

Changing from oral morphine to diamorphine injection

When patients are first changed over to a syringe driver, they will usually have been taking oral morphine beforehand. There is a table with suggested dosage conversion in the BNF (2008). The dose conversion stated in the BNF for a four-hourly dose is:

5 mg oral morphine = 1.25 – 2.5 mg sub-cutaneous diamorphine

This may vary according to the reference text used: some authors allow for the fact that starting a syringe driver usually indicates loss of control of pain and an automatic slight increase in dose is built in. When calculating the total dose of oral morphine, we must remember to add the total of the non-slow-release doses used for breakthrough pain as well as the regular slow-release doses.

Example: We will use the 2:1 ratio. A patient is taking morphine sulphate slow-release tablets 100 mg twice a day for pain and morphine sulphate non-slow-release tablets 30 mg about four times a day for breakthrough pain. You want to change to a syringe driver. What is the equivalent sub-cutaneous dose of diamorphine?

Step 1: Calculate the total daily dose of oral morphine.

Slow-release morphine: 100 mg twice a day   = 200 mg

Non-slow-release morphine: 30 mg four times a day = 120 mg

Total daily dose of morphine   = 320 mg

Step 2: Calculate the equivalent sub-cutaneous dose of diamorphine.

2 mg oral morphine = 1 mg sub-cutaneous diamorphine

Therefore a dose of 320 mg oral morphine is equivalent to:

$$320 \times \frac{1}{2} = 160 \text{ mg}$$

Test yourself with practice calculations

27. Calculate the contents of the following syringe driver in millilitres.

Diamorphine hydrochloride	50 mg (dissolved in 2ml water for injection)
Metoclopramide	40 mg
Levomepromazine	12.5 mg
Water for injection to	17 ml

This formulation has been checked for stability (Dickman et al. 2002).

28. A patient is taking 60 mg morphine sulphate slow-release tablets twice a day. What is the correct dose of oral morphine sulphate solution for breakthrough pain?
29. A patient is taking 15 mg of morphine sulphate solution every 4 hours regularly. What is the equivalent dose of slow-release morphine tablets to be taken every 12 hours?
30. A patient is taking 90 mg morphine sulphate slow-release tablets BD regularly and is needing about 4 × 30 mg breakthrough doses of oral morphine solution. Calculate the equivalent dose of diamorphine to use if the patient was converted to a syringe driver.

Answers

1. a. 1.5 kg × 1000 = 1500 g

    b. 37.5 mg × 1000 = 37500 micrograms

    c. 650 microgram ÷ 1000 = 0.65 mg

    d. 1750 ml ÷ 1000 = 1.75 L

    e. 0.95 L × 1000 = 950 ml

2. Total amount of ointment:

Face:	30 g
Both hands:	50 g
Scalp:	100 g
Both arms:	200 g
Both legs:	200 g
Trunk:	400 g
Groin:	25 g
Total:	1005 g

    Total amount in kilograms is $1005 \div 1000 = 1.005$ kg

3. Calculate the total daily dose of the drug in micrograms.

    150 micrograms $\times$ 25 = 3750 microgram

    Convert the total daily dose into milligrams

    3750 microgram $\div$ 1000 = 3.75 mg

4. Calculate how much fluid the patient will need in one day.

    30 ml $\times$ 65 = 1950 ml

    Convert the volume into litres.

    1950 ml $\div$ 1000 = 1.95 L

5. Calculate how much the patient will take in one day.

    20 ml $\times$ 4 = 80 ml

    Calculate how much the patient will need for 30 days.

    80 ml $\times$ 30 = 2400 ml

    Convert the volume into litres.

    2400 ml $\div$ 1000 = 2.4 L

6. Step 1: Work out what the ratio strength means.

    Potassium permanganate 1 in 10 000 = 1 g in 10 000 ml

    Step 2: Convert the strength of the solution to milligrams.

    $$1 \text{ g in } 10\,000 \text{ ml} = 1 \times 1000 \text{ mg in } 10\,000 \text{ ml}$$
    $$= 1000 \text{ mg in } 10\,000 \text{ ml}$$

    Step 3: Calculate how much potassium permanganate there is in 100 ml of the solution.

    $$\frac{100}{10\,000} \times 1000 = 10 \text{ mg}$$

7. Step 1: Work out what the percentage strength means in grams per 100 ml.

    Hydrogen peroxide 6% solution contains 6 g hydrogen peroxide in 100 ml solution.

    Step 2: Calculate how much hydrogen peroxide there is in 250 ml of the solution.

    $$\frac{250}{100} \times 6 = 15 \text{ g in } 250 \text{ ml}$$

8. You have levomepromazine injection 25 mg in 1 ml.
   Step 1: Calculate the volume of solution that contains 6.25 mg levomepromazine.

   $$\frac{6.25}{25} \times 1\,ml = 0.25\,ml$$

9. Step 1: Calculate the total dose of the drug.

   $$25\,mg \times 18 = 450\,mg$$

   Step 2: Calculate the volume of mixture that contains 450 mg.
   Mixture contains 200 mg in 5 ml.
   Therefore, the volume that contains 450 mg will be:

   $$\frac{450}{200} \times 5\,ml = 11.25\,ml$$

10. Step 1: Work out what the percentage strength means in grams per 100 ml.
    Lidocaine 2% injection contains 2 g lidocaine in 100 ml solution.
    Step 2: Convert the strength of solution to milligrams in 100 ml.

    $$2\,g \text{ in } 100\,ml = 2 \times 1000\,mg \text{ in } 100\,ml$$
    $$= 2000\,mg \text{ in } 100\,ml$$

    Step 3: Calculate the volume of lidocaine injection that will contain 100 mg.

    $$\frac{100}{2000} \times 100\,ml = 5\,ml$$

11. a. What is the ideal body weight for a male who is 185 cm tall?

    Male: Ideal body weight $= (0.9 \times \text{height in centimetres}) - 88 \text{ kg}$
    $$= (0.9 \times 185) - 88 \text{ kg}$$
    $$= (166.5) - 88 \text{ kg}$$
    $$= 78.5 \text{ kg}$$

    Note: remember to multiply the numbers in brackets before you subtract the 88 kg.

11. b. What is the ideal body weight for a female who is 150 cm tall?

    Female: Ideal body weight $= (0.9 \times \text{height in centimetres}) - 92 \text{ kg}$
    $$= (0.9 \times 150) - 92 \text{ kg}$$
    $$= (135) - 92 \text{ kg}$$
    $$= 43 \text{ kg}$$

12. Calculate the total daily dose.

    Daily dose at 0.8 ml/kg $=$ Patient's weight (kg) $\times$ Daily dose (ml/kg)
    $$= 16 \text{ kg} \times 0.8 \text{ ml/kg}$$
    $$= 12.8 \text{ ml per day}$$

Calculate the dose to be given three times a day.

$$= 12.8 \text{ ml} \div 3$$
$$= 4.267 \text{ ml}$$
$$= 4.3 \text{ ml (rounded up to a practical dose)}$$

13. Calculate the ideal body weight.

Female: Ideal body weight $= (0.9 \times \text{height in centimetres}) - 92 \text{ kg}$
$$= (0.9 \times 165) - 92 \text{ kg}$$
$$= 148.5 - 92 \text{ kg}$$
$$= 56.5 \text{ kg}$$

Calculate the total daily dose.

Total daily dose at 5mg/kg $=$ Patient's IBW (kg) $\times$ daily dose (mg/kg)
$$= 56.5 \text{ kg} \times 5 \text{ mg/kg}$$
$$= 282.5 \text{ mg}$$

Either calculate the dose to be given every eight hours:

$$= 282.5 \div 3$$
$$= 94.17 \text{ mg (rounded to 95mg)}$$

Or calculate the dose to be given every six hours:

$$= 282.5 \div 4$$
$$= 70.63 \text{ mg (rounded to 70 mg)}$$

Convert to a practical dose for administration to the patient:
If tobramycin injection contains 40 mg in 1 ml, the two doses above would equate to:

Either 95 mg every 8 hours $= \dfrac{95}{40} \times 1 \text{ ml} = 2.375 \text{ ml}$

Or 70 mg every 6 hours $= \dfrac{70}{40} \times 1 \text{ ml} = 1.75 \text{ ml}$

14. Weekly dose of cyclophosphamide $= 120 \text{ mg/m}^2 \times 1.95 \text{ m}^2$
$$= 234 \text{ mg}$$

15. 1 L saline over 12 hours $= 1000 \text{ ml}/12 = 83.3 \text{ ml/hr}$

83.3 ml/hr $= 83.3/60 = 1.39 \text{ ml/min}$

This could be rounded up to 1.4 ml/min

20 drops $= 1$ ml, therefore 1.4 ml $= 1.4 \times 20 = 28$ drops per minute.

Therefore the drip rate controller should be set so that it administers 28 drops in one minute.

16. 500 ml glucose 5% over 3 hours = 500/3 = 166.7 ml/hr

    166.7 ml/hr = 166.7/60 = 2.8 ml/min

    20 drops = 1 ml, therefore 2.8 ml = 2.8 × 20 = 56 drops per minute

    Therefore the drip rate controller should be set so that it administers 56 drops in one minute.

17. 2.5 mcg/kg/min for a 75 kg patient = 2.5 × 75 mcg/min = 187.5 mcg/min

    187.5 mcg/min = 187.5 × 60 mcg/hr = 11 250 mcg/hr

    Convert to milligram per hour: 1000 mcg = 1 mg

    Therefore: 11 250 mcg/hr = 11.25 mg/hr

    The solution contains 250 mg dobutamine in 500 ml saline. How much does it contain in 1 ml?

    $$250 \text{ mg in } 500 \text{ ml} = \frac{1 \text{ ml}}{500 \text{ ml}} \times 250 \text{ mg} = 0.5 \text{ mg in } 1 \text{ ml}$$

    What volume will contain 11.25 mg?

    11.25 mg / 0.5 mg × 1 ml = 22.5 ml/hr

    Therefore the pump should be set to administer 22.5 ml/hr.

18. 2 mcg/kg/min in a patient weighing 65 kg = 130 mcg/min

    130 mcg/min × 60 = 7800 mcg/hr

    Convert to milligram per hour: 1000 mcg = 1 mg

    Therefore: 7800 mcg = 7.8 mg

    The dopamine solution contains 800 mg in 500 ml. How much does it contain in 1 ml?

    $$\frac{1 \text{ ml}}{500 \text{ ml}} \times 800 \text{ mg} = 1.6 \text{ mg in } 1 \text{ ml}$$

    $$\frac{7.8 \text{ mg}}{1.6 \text{ mg}} \times 1 \text{ ml} = 4.875 \text{ ml/hr}$$

    Therefore the pump should be set to administer 4.88 ml/hr.

19. Loading dose:

    5 mg per kg × 65 kg = 325 mg over 20 mins in either normal saline or glucose 5% infusion

    Maintenance dose:

    500 mcg/kg/hr in a patient weighing 65 kg = 500 × 65 mcg/hr

    = 32 500 mcg/hr

    Convert to milligram per hour: = 32.5 mg/hr

    The solution contains 500 mg in 500 ml, or 1 mg in 1 ml.
    Therefore the maintenance infusion should be set at 32.5 ml/hr.

20. 65 kg × 2.5 mg/kg = 162.5 mg.

    When divided into two doses, this would theoretically be 81.25 mg twice daily. This dose could be rounded either up to 100 mg twice daily or down to 75 mg twice daily. In practice, the dose should be rounded down to 75 mg twice daily because this is closer to the calculated dose. The blood level of ciclosporin should then be checked and the dose adjusted for the individual patient.

21. What is the *cost per tablet* of each of these drugs (rounded to the nearest whole number)?

    Ibuprofen 400 mg   £2.24 = 224p/84 = 3 pence

    Diclofenac 50 mg   £1.79 = 179/84 = 2 pence

    Naproxen 500 mg   £1.65 = 165/28 = 6 pence

    What is the *cost per treatment day* of each of these drugs (rounded to the nearest whole number)?

    Ibuprofen 400 mg   3 pence × 3 a day = 9 pence

    Diclofenac 50 mg   2 pence × 3 a day = 6 pence

    Naproxen 500 mg   6 pence × 2 a day = 12 pence

    What is the *cost per treatment course* of each of these drugs?

    Ibuprofen 400 mg   9p pence × 28 days = 252 pence = £2.52

    Diclofenac 50 mg   6 pence × 28 days = 118 pence = £1.68

    Naproxen 500 mg   12 pence × 28 days = 336 pence = £3.36

22. What is the cost per treatment day of each of these antacids (rounded to one decimal place)?

    Cost per ml of liquid:

    Gastrocote   £2.67 = 267p/500 = 0.5p per ml

    Gaviscon Advance   £2.70 = 270p/500 = 0.5p per ml

    Peptac   £2.16 = 216p/250 = 0.9p per ml

    Dosage per day:

    Gastrocote (15×4) = 60 ml

    Gaviscon Advance (10×4) = 40 ml

    Peptac (10×4) = 40 ml

    Cost per day of liquid:

    Gastrocote   0.5p per ml × 60 ml = 30 p

    Gaviscon Advance   0.5p per ml × 40 ml = 20 p

    Peptac   0.9p per ml × 40 ml = 36 p

a. What is the cost per treatment course of each of these antacids?

Gastrocote	30p × 28 days	= £8.40
Gaviscon Advance	20p × 28 days	= £5.60
Peptac	36p × 28 days	= £10.08

23.

Drug	Half-life	Time to steady state plasma concentration (4 to 5 times half-life)
Paracetamol	2 hours	8–10 hrs
Indomethacin	2.4 hours	9.6–12 hrs
Meloxicam	20 hours	80–100 hrs
Piroxicam	48 hours	192–240 hrs

24. After one half-life (eight hours), the theophylline level will have reduced by half.

28 mg/L ÷ 2 = 14 mg/L.

This lies within the reference range of 10–15 mg/L.

25. Step 1: Phenytoin sodium capsule 100 mg = phenyton liquid 90 mg.

$$\text{Step 2 : phenytoin sodium capsule} \left(3 \times 100\,\text{mg}\right) + \left(1 \times 50\,\text{mg}\right)$$
$$= \text{phenytoin liquid} \left(3 \times 90\text{mg}\right) + \left(1 \times 45\,\text{mg}\right)$$
$$= \text{phenytoin liquid } 315\,\text{mg}$$

Step 3: Phenytoin liquid contains 30 mg phenytoin in 5 ml. Therefore what volume contains 315 mg?

$$\frac{315\,\text{mg}}{30\,\text{mg}} \times 5\,\text{ml} = 52.5\,\text{ml}$$

26. Step 1: total daily dose of carbamazepine = 400 mg × 2 = 800 mg

Step 2: convert 800 mg orally to the equivalent in suppositories

100 mg orally = 125 mg rectally

Therefore, 800 mg orally = $\left(8 \times 125\,\text{mg}\right)$ rectally

$$= 1000\,\text{mg}$$

Step 3: No more than 250 mg can be given at a time by the rectal route. Therefore a rectal dose of 1000 mg must be given as 250 mg four times a day.

27. Step 1: Calculate the amount of each ingredient.
Diamorphine = 50 mg in 2 ml water for injections (as stated).
Metoclopramide injection contains 10 mg in 2 ml.
Therefore, metoclopramide 40 mg = 8 ml.
Levomepromazine injection contains 25 mg in 1 ml.
Therefore, levomepromazine 12.5 mg = 0.5 ml.
Step 2: Calculate the volume of water for injection required.

Total volume of the final solution is stated as 17 ml.

Therefore the amount of water for injection will be:

$$(17 \text{ ml} - 2 \text{ ml} - 8 \text{ ml} - 0.5 \text{ ml}) = 6.5 \text{ ml}$$

Therefore the patient would need a supply of 10 ml ampoules of water for injection.

28. Step 1: Calculate the total daily dose of morphine.

    $$60 \text{ mg} \times 2 = 120 \text{ mg}$$

    Step 2: Calculate the breakthrough dose of morphine.

    $$120 \text{ mg} \div 6 = 20 \text{ mg}$$

    A dose of 20 mg non-slow-release morphine should be prescribed, usually taken every four hours or more often according to patient need.

29. Step 1: Calculate the total daily dose of non-slow-release morphine.

    $$15 \text{ mg every 4 hours} = 15 \text{ mg} \times 6 = 90 \text{ mg}$$

    Step 2: Calculate the equivalent dose of slow-release morphine.

    $$90 \text{ mg} \div 2 = 45 \text{ mg twice a day}$$

30. Step 1: total daily morphine $= (90 \text{ mg} \times 2) + (30 \text{ mg} \times 4) = 300 \text{ mg}$

    Step 2: sub-cutaneous dose of diamorphine $= 300 \text{ mg} \div 2 = 150 \text{ mg}$

References

Bauman, J. (2002). Antiarrhythmic drugs. pp 297–323. In Anderson, P., Knoben, J., Troutman, W. (eds). *Handbook of Clinical Drug Data*. New York: McGraw-Hill Medical Publishing Division.

Bonner, M., Wright, D., George, B. (2001). *Practical Pharmaceutical Calculations*. Newbury: Petroc Press (LibraPharm Limited).

British National Formulary no 56. (2008). London: BMJ Publishing Group Ltd and RPS Publishing.

Courtenay, M., Griffiths, M. (eds) (2010). *Medication Safety: An Essential Guide*. Cambridge: Cambridge University Press.

Department of Health (2001). *National Guidance on Intrathecal Chemotherapy*. HSC 2001/022. London: Department of Health.

Department of Health (2003). *Updated National Guidance on the Safe Administration of Intrathecal Chemotherapy*. HSC 2003/010. London: Department of Health.

Dickman, A., Littlewood, C., Varga, J. (2002). *The Syringe Driver: Continuous Subcutaneous Infusions in Palliative Care*. Oxford: Oxford University Press.

DuBois, D., DuBois, E.F. (1916). Cited in Jones, P.R., Wilkinson, S., Davies, P.S. (1985). A revision of body surface area estimations. *Eur J Appl Physiol Occup Physiol* 53(4): 376–379.

Electronic Medicines Compendium (2007). SPC cyclophosphamide. http://emc.medicines.org.uk

Electronic Medicines Compendium (2009). SPC vincristine sulphate 1mg/ml injection. http://emc.medicines.org.uk

Lesar, S. (1998). Errors in the use of medication dosage equations. *Arch Pediatr Adolesc Med* 152(4): 340–344.

MacLean, F., Macintyre, J., McDade, J. et al. (2003). Dose banding of chemotherapy in the Edinburgh Cancer Centre. *Pharm J 270*: 691–693.

Marshik, P. (2002). Antihistamines. pp 790–803. In Anderson, P., Knoben, J., Troutman, W. (eds) *Handbook of Clinical Drug Data*. New York: McGraw-Hill Medical Publishing Division.

Mercier, R.C. (2002a). Aminoglycosides. pp 55–61. In Anderson, P., Knoben, J., Troutman, W. (eds) *Handbook of Clinical Drug Data*. New York: McGraw-Hill Medical Publishing Division.

Mercier, R.C. (2002b). Beta-lactams. pp 126–158. In Anderson, P., Knoben, J., Troutman, W. (eds) *Handbook of Clinical Drug Data*. New York: McGraw-Hill Medical Publishing Division.

National Patient Safety Agency (2007). *Patient Safety Alert 20: Promoting Safer Use of Injectable Medicines*. London: National Patient Safety Agency.

National Patient Safety Agency (2008). *Rapid Response Report NPSA/2008/RRR04. Using Vinca Alkaloid Minibags (Adult/Adolescent Units)*. http://www.npsa.nhs.uk/patientsafety/alerts-and-directives/rapidrr

National Prescribing Centre (2001). *Maintaining Competency in Prescribing: an Outline Framework to Help Nurse Prescribers*. http://www.npc.co.uk/prescribers/resources/maint_comp_prescribing_nurs.pdf

National Prescribing Centre (2004). Maintaining Competency in Prescribing: an Outline Framework to Help Allied Health Professional Supplementary Prescribers. http://www.npc.co.uk/prescribers/resources/maintain_comp_prescribing.pdf

National Prescribing Centre (2006). *Maintaining Competency in Prescribing: an Outline Framework to Help Pharmacist Prescribers* (second edition). http://www.npc.co.uk/prescribers/resources/competency_framework_oct_2006.pdf

Nursing and Midwifery Council (2004). *Standards of Proficiency for Pre-registration Nursing Education*. http://www.nmc-uk.org/aFrameDisplay.aspx?DocumentID=328&Keyword=

Nursing and Midwifery Council (2006). *Standards of Proficiency for Nurse and Midwife Prescribers*. http://www.nmc-uk.org/aArticle.aspx?ArticleID=2021

Setter, S., Baker, D. (2002). Nonsteroidal anti-inflammatory drugs. pp 16–30. In Anderson, P., Knoben, J., Troutman, W. (eds). *Handbook of Clinical Drug Data*. New York: McGraw-Hill Medical Publishing Division.

Smith, J. (2004). *Building a Safer NHS for Patients: Improving Medication Safety*. London: Department of Health.

Stimmel, G. (2002). Antidepressants. pp 444–459. In Anderson, P., Knoben, J., Troutman, W. (eds) *Handbook of Clinical Drug Data*. New York: McGraw-Hill Medical Publishing Division.

Wang, Y., Moss, J., Thisted, R. (1992). Predictors of body surface area. *J Clin Anesth* 4(1): 4–10.

Chapter 13

Prescribing in practice: how it works

Polly Buchanan

Williams (1997) cites that at least 25% of the total population of the UK have a skin complaint, of which 19% will consult their GP. Therefore, caring for patients with dermatological conditions represents a significant workload for health professionals in primary care. Future dermatology services are aimed at improving dermatology services within primary care (DoH 2006) and reducing the waiting times for patients to be seen in secondary care (DoH 2008). This has already resulted in the development of nurse-led clinics in primary care for patients with chronic inflammatory skin disease (Bowcock and Bailey 2002; Mateos 2003; Page et al. 2009; Rolfe 2002a). Eczematous conditions, psoriasis and acne represent the three main chronic relapsing diseases which can be managed more effectively in a primary care setting (Page et al. 2009).

Recent legislative changes surrounding the prescription of medications will enable nurse-led clinics and pharmacy services to complement GP and secondary care dermatology services (Bowman 2000; DoH 1999; 2000; 2002; 2003; Medicines Control Agency 2002). For example, some of the topical and systemic medications used in dermatology are now available for nurses to prescribe independently. Furthermore, the advent of supplementary prescribing has meant that both nurses and pharmacists are able to prescribe from the *British National Formulary* (BNF 2009) for patients with dermatological conditions through the use of Clinical Management Plans (CMPs).

The competency frameworks such as those developed by the National Prescribing Centre (NPC 2003), the Nursing and Midwifery Council (NMC 2003) and NHS Scotland (NHS Education for Scotland 2003) have enabled practitioners to acquire general prescribing competencies and those specific to dermatology in order for them to work competently in the role of prescriber. These include competencies in relation to:

- Clinical assessment of the patient's skin.
- Assessment of the patient's physiological, psychological and emotional response to a given dermatological diagnosis.
- Assessment of the patient's response to therapeutic interventions and so the implementation of effective and safe therapeutic interventions.
- Provision of support and information regarding skin care.

This chapter describes how independent and supplementary prescribing can be used by non-medical prescribers in the treatment management of patients with dermatological conditions. It is hoped that readers will be provided with valuable insights with regard to how these modes of prescribing can be used to enhance patient care in other areas of practice and optimise the role of the non-medical practitioners involved in prescribing.

Skin care

We are exposed to the concept of skin care on a daily basis. The cosmetic industry encourages everyone to care for their skin to aid attractiveness and prevent ageing. Many cosmetics and beauty products are designed specifically for skin. Fashion and beauty industries have made our expectations of having beautiful skin integral to our psyche. The 'look' of our skin affects our self-esteem. Therefore, it is important that healthcare professionals involved in caring for patients with skin-related disease, as well as having a basic understanding of the anatomy and physiology of normal skin and knowledge of common dermatoses, also appreciate the effects of overt skin disease on self-image and how important it is to provide adequate care for these individuals (Papadopoulos and Bor 1999).

Prescribing for patients with dermatological conditions

The skin is the largest vital organ of the body and can be effectively treated via the transcutaneous route. Therefore, the majority of medications used in dermatology are topical. The advent

Table 13.1. Skin conditions for which nurse prescribers are able to prescribe (BNF 2009)

Abrasions
Acne
Actinic keratoses
Boil/carbuncle
Burn/scald
Blistering conditions
Candidiasis
Chronic skin ulcer
Dermatitis (atopic, contact, seborrhoeic)
Dermatophytosis of the skin (ringworm)
Drug eruptions
Herpes labialis
Impetigo
Insect bites/stings
Lacerations
Juvenile plantar dermatoses
Nappy rash
Pediculosis (head lice)
Pityriasis
Pruritus in chickenpox
Rosacea
Scabies
Urticaria
Warts (including verrucas)

of independent prescribing has further facilitated therapeutic interventions for a number of dermatological conditions by non-medical prescribers (see Table 13.1).

Major factors influencing the use of topical and systemic medications in dermatology

The greatest benefits of topical medications are the safety profiles (low potential for systemic absorption/toxicity), efficacy profiles (good transcutaneous absorption), minimal side effects and cost-effectiveness. However, the greatest disadvantages of topical medications used in dermatology relate to the odour, the appearance, the consistency, the frequency of application and staining of skin, hair, furniture and clothes. These disadvantages are incongruent with patient concordance.

For example, patients with psoriasis who are self-caring for their skin at home frequently report difficulties in using tar-based or anthralin-based preparations. These medications are effective if used with support and education, although it takes a very dedicated and motivated patient to use these products in the moderate and long term due to the staining of skin, clothes and furniture. Consideration and discussion of other less 'messy' topical preparations for psoriasis, such as vitamin D analogues, corticosteroids and retinoids, as other treatment options will demand further patient education. Therefore, before the patient is able to choose or agree to the appropriate medication, they require an understanding of such factors as the side effects and the possibility of tachyphylaxis with long-term usage.

If the prescriber is to achieve patient concordance and thus clinical effectiveness, a good understanding of basic pharmacology and its application to the treatment management of these patients is essential. This includes an understanding of how each medicine exerts its effect, and how individual patient differences alter this effect. This will enable decisions to be made about the route of administration of a drug, the dose and frequency, contraindications and adverse effects.

Furthermore, seeking a cure is not a viable outcome for chronic relapsing skin disease, such as psoriasis or eczema. Dermatological patients frequently report that the most difficult aspect of their skin condition is learning to live with it (Buchanan 2001; McGuckin 2003). It is therefore essential that the practitioner feels confident to help the patient manage their skin during a lifetime, reducing the severity of relapses and extending the periods of remission. Being an educator, advisor, assessor and auditor are important components within the prescriber's remit role. This can be achieved if the patient's concerns, lifestyle, age, abilities and individual coping strategies are understood by the practitioner.

Patients with chronic relapsing skin disease have generally developed a deep understanding of their condition (Titman 2001), i.e. how it affects their life and which treatment regimens are effective for them. If practitioners are to identify and select the most appropriate medication for the patient, assessment should include the physical, psychological, emotional, social and spiritual aspects of the patient's life and how the disease affects them. This will enable the patient to become a partner in their care and so greatly influence how they use the medications prescribed.

Information and advice provided by the prescriber to the patient represent the most important factors that influence the use of topical medication (Gradwell 2001). Inadequate information and support during a treatment programme often result in misunderstanding, disillusionment and poor concordance by the patient (Davis 2002; Titman 2001; Wilson et al. 2009). The length of time for medications to take effect (often weeks) and the nature of topical formulations further compound the problem of poor concordance.

Rotational therapy, whereby topical treatments are alternated (including treatment holidays), is advocated in the management of psoriasis by the British Association of Dermatologists. This reduces the likelihood of tachyphylaxis and promotes patient concordance. Rotation of topical therapies every 6–12 weeks can aid the therapeutic effect (AAD 2003; Ali 2003; BAD 2009).

The treatment management of acne vulgaris (discussed below) is used to demonstrate how effective prescribing can enhance patient care.

Acne vulgaris

Acne vulgaris is an inflammatory condition which affects the pilosebaceous units of the skin. The face, neck, shoulders, chest and back are often affected and it is extremely common during adolescence and early adulthood. Acne vulgaris is characterised by an increase in sebum production, presence of open and closed comedones, an increase in the *Propionibacterium acnes (P. acnes)* organism in the gland duct, an increase in free fatty acids and inflammation around the sebaceous gland (Buxton 1993). The disease may include a variety of skin lesions from non-inflammatory comedones to inflammatory papules and pustules. Severe acne may also comprise cysts and scars.

The treatment management of acne vulgaris

Prescribing for acne depends on severity and the psychological impact the condition has on the patient (NICE 2000). Even mild acne can have such a devastating effect on the patient's self-esteem that active medical intervention is necessary. Moderate to severe acne requires early and sustained medical intervention to prevent scarring and control exacerbations (Papadopoulos and Bor 1999). Management strategies relate to the pathology of the disease and incorporate anticomedonal, antimicrobial and antibacterial agents, and anti-androgen preparations (Cunningham 2000; Rolfe 2002b).

Topical retinoids, topical antimicrobials, topical antibiotics and systemic antibiotics are preparations used to treat mild to moderate comedonal and inflammatory acne vulgaris (BAD 2004; Global Alliance 2003). General Sales List (GSL) and Pharmacist Only (P) acne medications can be recommended to the patient and supplied by pharmacists. For supplementary prescribers, CMPs are an essential component of prescribing documentation. Figure 13.1 outlines a CMP that might be used for the management of mild to moderate acne.

Treatment complications

Complications that may arise when treating patients with acne vulgaris surround poor patient concordance, i.e. intermittent application, antibiotic resistance and irritation.

For example, managing the comedonal component of acne is fundamental in the treatment management of this condition. Comedones and micro-comedones are the precursor lesions to the inflammatory papules and pustules of acne. Therefore, anticomedonal therapies are an essential component of the overall treatment. Topical naphthoic acid derivatives and retinoids are the recommended groups of drugs for comedonal acne. They are indicated for active treatment and maintenance therapy and can be used as a monotherapy for uncomplicated comedonal acne, but most often combination therapy is indicated with antimicrobial agents or antibacterials. Support and advice is essential when prescribing topical retinoids due to the irritation these preparations can cause. Naphthoic acid is less irritant to the skin compared to other topical retinoids. The irritant potential of the medication needs to be

Name of Patient: MISS Y	Patient medication sensitivities/allergies: None known

Patient identification e.g. ID number, date of birth: 21/2/85	

Independent Prescriber(s): DR G	Supplementary Prescriber(s) Sister A

Condition(s) to be treated Acne vulgaris	Aim of treatment To reduce, control and prevent comedonal, seborrhoea and inflammatory components of acne with minimal side effects. To reduce scarring.

Medicines that may be prescribed by SP:

Preparation MILD comedonal acne	Indication	Dose schedule	Specific indications for referral back to the IP
1.Topical Naphthoic acid or retinoids (+ inflammatory lesions)	Reduction and control of comedonal lesions and inflammatory lesions in mild to moderate acne	*As detailed in:* *BNF Section 13.6.1 topical preparations for acne*	
2. Topical antimicrobials Benzoyl peroxide +/- naphthoic acid/ retinoids; antibiotics	Reduction and control of comedonal and inflammatory lesions in mild to moderate acne	*As above*	*Diagnosis in doubt*
MODERATE (inflammatory papules and pustules)	Reduction and control of inflammatory acne of moderate severity	*BNF Section 13.6.2 oral antibacterials for acne*	*Failure to respond to treatment*
+/-3. Systemic antibiotics +/- topical benzoyl +/topical naphthoic acid +/- topical retinoids +/-4. Systemic anti-androgen	*Reduction and control of seborrhoeic component in moderate acne*	*As above*	

Guidelines or protocols supporting Clinical Management Plan:

Consult local formulary guidelines for first choice of topical and systemic drugs (practitioner would be required to reference these guidelines in the CMP)

BNF prescribing guidelines

British Association of Dermatologists Guidelines

Frequency of review and monitoring by:

Supplementary prescriber As indicated by response 1-3 monthly	Supplementary prescriber and independent prescriber No less than 6 monthly

Process for reporting ADRs:

Yellow Card system. Verbal and written reporting by SP to IP

Shared record to be used by IP and SP:

Nurse-led clinic documentation (Integrated Care Pathway and clinical assessment records) as well as computerised patient records within Surgery or Practice

Agreed by independent prescriber(s)	Date	Agreed by supplementary prescriber(s)	Date	Date agreed with patient/carer

Figure 13.1 CMP for mild to moderate acne

explained to the patient with mention of mild scaling, dryness and erythema. Advice on how applications can be titrated to reduce side effects should also be provided.

Antibacterial agents help control colonisation of *P. acnes*, the organism responsible for mediating the inflammatory response in acne. Resistance of *P. acnes* is increasing, therefore prescribing of antibiotics is restricted to cases which are unresponsive to antibacterial agents. Prolonged or continuous courses of topical antibiotics encourage resistance. Therefore, courses should be adequate to treat the condition and then discontinued. Topical antibiotics should be continued for at least six months. Systemic antibiotics are reserved for cases where topical medications are ineffective. A course of tetracycline antibiotics should demonstrate a response by three months with continued effect between four and six months. Treatment can be continued as long as clinical improvement continues. If there is no adequate response at three months, another systemic antibiotic should be considered. It is vital that patients are provided with the appropriate information about their condition and the antibacterial therapy in order that patient concordance is increased and the risk of antibacterial resistance is reduced.

As already highlighted, information and advice provided by the prescriber to the patient represent the most important factors that influence the use of topical medication (Gradwell 2001). As prescribing requires consent by the patient for the management partnership to go ahead, nurse prescribing, with its strong focus on ongoing education, provides an excellent framework for the treatment management of this condition and should improve patient adherence to treatment regimes.

Conclusion

This chapter has discussed some of the key issues involved in the prescription of medicines for patients with skin disease and specifically acne vulgaris. Some of the major influencing factors in the use of topical and systemic medications for these conditions have been outlined. Although nurses are able to prescribe independently for a number of dermatological conditions, supplementary prescribing has enabled both nurses and pharmacists to prescribe for many additional skin diseases.

Information and advice represent the most important factors influencing the use of topical medication by patients with dermatological conditions. Nurse prescribing, with its strong focus on education and support, provides an ideal framework within which to prescribe medicines for these patients.

References

Ali, O. (2003). The management of psoriasis. Part one: tachyphylaxis. *Br J Dermatol Nursing* 7(3): 6–7.

American Academy of Dermatologists (2003). Consensus statement on psoriasis therapies. *J Am Acad Derm* 49: 897–899.

Bowcock, S., Bailey, K. (2002). The introduction of nurse led clinics in dermatology. *Br J Dermatol Nursing* 1(4): 22.

Bowman, J. (2000). Nurse prescribing in a day-care dermatology unit. *Professional Nurse* 15(9): 573–577.

British Association of Dermatologists (2004a). Acne Guidelines. www.bad.org.uk/doctors/guidelines/acne.asp

British Association of Dermatologists (2004b). Acne. www.bad.org.uk/patients/disease/acne

British National Formulary (2009). London: BMJ Group and RPS Publishing.

Buchanan, P.J. (2001). Behaviour modification: a nursing approach for young children with atopic eczema. *Dermatology Nursing* 13(1): 15–25.

Buxton, P.K. (1993). *ABC of Dermatology*. London: BMJ Publishing Group.

Cunningham, M. (2000). Effective acne treatment. *Br J Dermatol Nursing* 4(4): 12–15.

Davis, R. (2002). Caring for the skin at home. In: Penzer, R. (ed). *Nursing Care of the Skin*. Oxford: Butterworth Heinemann.

Department of Health (1999). *Review of Prescribing, Supply and Administration of Medicines. Final Report* (Crown report). London: DoH.

Department of Health (2000). *The NHS Plan: A Plan for Investment. A Plan for Reform*. London: The Stationery Office.

Department of Health (2002). *Extending Independent Nurse Prescribing Within the NHS in England. A Guide for Implementation*. London: DoH.

Department of Health (2003). *Supplementary Prescribing by Nurses and Pharmacists within the NHS in England. A Guide for Implementation*. London: DoH.

Gradwell, C. (2001). How to… meet the educational needs of a dermatology patient. *Br J Dermatol Nursing* 5(4): 12–13.

Mateos, M. (2002). The health visitor role in setting up a nurse-led eczema clinic. *Br J Dermatol Nursing* 1(4): 6–8.

McGuckin, F. (2003). My journey with psoriasis. *Br J Dermatol Nursing* 7(3): 14–15.

Medicines Control Agency (2002). *Proposals for Supplementary Prescribing by Nurses and Pharmacists and Proposed Amendments to the Prescription Only Medicines (Human Use) Order 1997*. London: DoH.

National Institute of Clinical Excellence (2000). *GP Referral Practice: A Guide to Appropriate Referral from General to Specialist Services*. London: NICE.

NHS Education for Scotland (2003). *Caring for People with Dermatology Conditions: A Core Curriculum*. Edinburgh: Quality Assuring Continuing Professional Development.

Nursing and Midwifery Council (2003). QA factsheet D6. www.nmc-uk.org/nmc/main / qa/docs/QA-c2003pdf

Papadopoulos, L., Bor, R. (1999). *Psychological Approaches to Dermatology*. Leicester: British Psychological Society.

Rolfe, G. (2002a). A nurse-led acne, psoriasis and eczema initiative in Northants. *Br J Dermatol Nursing* 1(4): 18–20.

Rolfe, G. (2002b). Nursing role for acne in primary care. *Br J Dermatol Nursing* 6(3): 9–11.

Titman, P. (2001). Understanding the stresses on mothers of children with eczema. *Br J Dermatol Nursing* 5(4): 7–9.

Williams, H. (1997). Dermatology. In: Stevens, A., Raftery, J. (eds). *Health Care Needs Assessment: The Epidemiologically Based Needs Assessment Reviews* (second edition). Oxford: Dadcliffe Medical Press.

Chapter 1

Minimising the risk of prescribing error

Gillian Cavell

Preventable medication errors occur at all stages of the medicines use process. Prescribing is no exception to this.

Prescription is the first stage in the medicines use process and prescribing errors are possibly the most serious of all types of medication errors. Unless a prescribing error is detected by another person involved in medicine use, such as the pharmacist dispensing the medicine, the nurse administering the medicine or the patient for whom the medicine was prescribed, incorrect medicines will be taken or given, with the risk of harm. The extent to which a prescribing error causes harm will depend on the drug prescribed, the magnitude of the error if it is a dosing error, the number of doses of the incorrect prescription the patient receives, the clinical status of the patient exposed to the error and the setting in which the error occurs. The same error in two different patients can have very different outcomes.

Traditionally only doctors and dentists could prescribe medicines. Now pharmacists, nurses and allied health professionals are extending their patient care roles and prescribing either as supplementary prescribers in partnership with independent prescribers or independently in their own right. These new prescribers will be vulnerable to the same systemic causes of prescribing error as traditional prescribers.

This chapter describes prescribing errors, their causes and actions to be taken to minimise the risk of prescribing error.

Definitions

The published definition of a prescribing error and the types of errors which fulfil that definition are useful in helping us to understand how errors occur and how they can be prevented:

> A clinically meaningful prescribing error occurs when, as a result of a prescribing decision or prescription writing process there is an unintentional significant (1) reduction in the probability of treatment being timely and effective or (2) increase in the risk of harm when compared with generally accepted practice (Dean et al. 2000).

Prescribing errors can either be as a result of errors in decision making or as a result of miscommunication during the prescription writing process.

Errors in decision making can occur as a result of lack of knowledge of the patient and their clinical status, or lack of knowledge of the drug being prescribed.

Types of prescribing error

Errors in decision making

Prescription inappropriate for the patient concerned

- Prescribing a drug for a patient for whom, as a result of a co-existing clinical decision, that drug is contraindicated.
- Prescribing a drug to which the patient has a documented clinically significant allergy.
- Not taking into account a potentially significant drug interaction.
- Prescribing a drug in a dose that, according to the *British National Formulary* or data sheet recommendations, is inappropriate for the patient's renal function.
- Prescription of a drug in a dose below (or above) that recommended for the patient's clinical condition.
- Prescribing a drug with a narrow therapeutic index, in a dose predicted to give serum levels significantly above the desired therapeutic range.
- Prescribing a drug with a narrow therapeutic index, in a dose predicted to give serum levels significantly below the desired therapeutic range.
- Not altering a dose following steady state serum levels significantly outside the desired therapeutic range.
- Continuing a drug in the event of a clinically significant adverse drug reaction.
- Prescribing two drugs for the same indication when only one of the drugs is necessary.
- Prescribing a drug for which there is no indication for the patient.

Pharmaceutical issues

- Prescribing a drug to be given by intravenous infusion in a diluent that is incompatible with the drug prescribed.
- Prescribing a drug to be infused via an intravenous peripheral line in a concentration greater than that recommended for peripheral administration.

Errors in prescription writing

Failure to communicate essential information

- Prescribing a drug, dose or route that is not intended.
- Writing illegibly.
- Writing a drug's name using abbreviations or other non-standard nomenclature.
- Writing an ambiguous medication order.
- Prescribing 'one tablet' of a drug where more than one strength is available.
- Omission of the route of administration for a drug that can be given by more than one route.
- Prescribing a drug to be given by intermittent intravenous infusion, without specifying the duration over which it is to be infused.
- Omission of the prescriber's signature.

Transcription error

- On admission to hospital, unintentionally not prescribing a drug that the patient was taking prior to their admission.

- Continuing a GP's prescribing error when writing a patient's drug chart on admission to hospital.
- Transcribing a medication order incorrectly when rewriting a patient's drug chart.
- Writing milligrams when micrograms was intended.
- Writing a prescription for discharge medication that unintentionally deviates from the medication prescribed on the inpatient drug chart.
- On admission to hospital, writing a medication order that unintentionally deviates from the patient's pre-admission prescription.

Many factors can contribute to prescribing error and awareness of the conditions that may result in error will enable prescribers to manage the risks in their own practice.

Lookalike and soundalike drug names

Practitioners have no control over the names given to medicines. All medicines have three names: a chemical name used by researchers but not usually used in clinical practice; a generic name created for a drug substance when it is marketed; and a brand name which is the trade-marked name given to the drug by the company that manufactures it.

Drugs belonging to the same pharmacological class

Generic names often include a stem of letters which indicate the pharmacological class to which the drug belongs. For example, monoclonal antibodies include the stem 'mab', while COX-2 inhibitors used in the treatment of rheumatoid and osteoarthritis include the stem 'coxib'. These common stems immediately introduce the risk of error due to drug name confusion and the risk is increased if drugs are available in similar dosage forms or in similar strengths.

Drugs manufactured by the same company

Brand or trade names for products manufactured by the same company may also look similar, especially where different formulations of the same product are manufactured.

Xalatan® eye drops, manufactured by Pharmacia, contain latanoprost. Pharmacia also manufacture eye drops containing a combination of latanoprost and timolol, called Xalacom®. The 'Xala' stem at the beginning of the drug name increases the risk of confusion between these two products. The drug names also contain the same number of letters and if poorly written can easily be confused.

The brand names of potassium chloride and sodium chloride tablets are Slow-K® and Slow Sodium®. Because of the prefix 'Slow' these products are easily confused. Similarly Sando-K® and Sandocal® may be confused.

Unrelated drugs containing similar strings of letters can be confused particularly if the similarities are in the first syllable of the drug name. As well as looking similar when written down, these drugs are also likely to appear next to one another in computerised drug dictionaries, increasing the likelihood of mis-selection errors. The Institute of Safe Medication Practices in the USA publishes a list of drug name pairs which are known to have been associated with medication error (ISMP 2005). Although this list includes American drug names, many are common to drug names used in the UK.

In the UK the National Patient Safety Agency (NPSA) has not published an equivalent comprehensive list of drug names which have been confused but gives the examples listed in Table 14.1 (NPSA 2007).

Table 14.1 Examples of pairs of drugs which have been confused in reports to the NPSA (2007)

vinblast**ine**	**vin**crist**ine**
cefotax**ime**	**cef**urox**ime**
morphine	dia**morphine**
a**drenaline**	**a**miodar**one**
hydroxy**zine**	**hydr**ala**zine**
amiodarone	**a**llopurinol
prostacyc**lin**	**prosta**gland**in**
bisacodyl	**bis**oprolol

Prescription writing standards

The prescription is the means of communicating the decision to treat a patient with a medicine to pharmacists dispensing medicines in primary and secondary care, and to nurses administering medicines in hospitals.

In the UK many prescriptions issued from general practice surgeries are generated from computerised prescribing systems. However, in hospitals, computerised prescribing systems are less well developed and the majority of prescriptions for inpatients and outpatients are handwritten.

Illegible handwriting on prescriptions is a well recognised source of medication error. Misinterpretation of a poorly written prescription can result in wrong drug, wrong dose, wrong frequency and wrong route errors. Drug doses may be delayed if the prescriber needs to be contacted to clarify the prescription. Prescribers themselves may not be aware that their handwriting is not legible as they will know their own intentions. Whether your own handwriting is legible to another person is difficult to determine as legibility is subjective and depends on the reader's own knowledge of drugs, the patient and the prescriber's intentions.

Check the legibility of your own handwriting

- In your normal handwriting write down the names of five drugs you will expect to prescribe.
- Ask a non-medically trained friend to transcribe the drug names.
- If the transcription is accurate then your handwriting is legible.

Community pharmacists dispensing prescriptions may not know the patient they are dispensing for and may not be aware of the patient's diagnosis or the prescriber's intentions. What is dispensed will be determined by the accuracy of the prescription and the pharmacist's interpretation of the prescription.

A patient died after taking the wrong medicine which was dispensed by a pharmacist from an illegible prescription. The prescriber intended the patient to receive 20 mg Isordil (isosorbide mononitrate) every six hours to treat angina. The prescription was misread by the pharmacist as Plendil (felodipine), which he dispensed at the same dose. The usual maximum daily dose of felodipine is 10 mg once a day. A day after taking the felodipine the patient had a heart attack and subsequently died. The doctor who wrote the illegible prescription and the

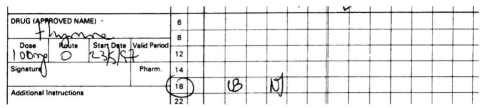

Figure 14.1 Illegible prescription leading to 'wrong drug' error

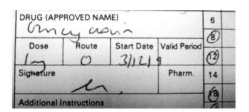

Figure 14.2 Unidentifiable prescription

pharmacist who dispensed the felodipine without questioning the dose were each ordered to pay compensation to the patient's family (Charatan 1999).

Misspelling a drug name can result in misinterpretation of a prescription. The prescription for a 100 mg dose of a drug in Figure 14.1 was misinterpreted resulting in the patient receiving the wrong drug.

The first three letters of the drug name clearly read 'thy' and the last two letters look like 'ne'. The middle is ambiguous. The drug name was interpreted as thyroxine and it was assumed that the prescriber intended the patient to receive 100 micrograms, not 100 mg as prescribed in the dose section of the chart. As a result, the patient was given thyroxine which was not indicated. The prescriber actually intended the patient to receive thiamine 100 mg daily which was omitted. Note also that it appears that on one occasion the patient received no dose, possibly because the nurse administering the drug did not feel that the prescription was safe.

The prescription in Figure 14.2 is assumed to read gancyclovir (ganciclovir) but the dose appears to be 1 mg. Again the patient missed doses as the drug name could not be interpreted and the dose did not correspond to the drug that was assumed to be required. (Note: oral ganciclovir is no longer available as it has been superceded by valganciclovir which is a pro-drug of ganciclovir.)

Abbreviations

Prescription writing guidance in the BNF states that 'the names of drugs and preparations should be written clearly and not abbreviated' (BNF 2008). The full approved name of the drug should always be used to avoid misinterpretation.

As well as misinterpretation of abbreviations for drug names, errors have occurred when abbreviations for dose units have been used. Again the BNF gives guidance on this and states: '"Micrograms" and "nanograms" should not be abbreviated. Similarly "units" should not be abbreviated.'

The abbreviation 'mcg' for micrograms may be misinterpreted as 'mg' (milligrams). This is unlikely to result in error with oral medicines as the size of the error would result in the patient requiring hundreds of tablets to give the required dose, an error that is likely to be spotted by even the most inexperienced pharmacist or nurse. However, misinterpretation may result in a dosing error in paediatrics where the size of doses based on body weight can vary much more widely.

Of more concern is abbreviation of the word unit, which can be written as 'u' or 'iu', as described in the next section.

Dose units

Drug doses are usually expressed in the amount of active drug in a dose unit, e.g. micrograms, milligrams, grams for solid dosage forms and milligrams or grams per unit volume for liquids, e.g. mg/ml or grams/5 ml. Doses should always be described as the amount of active ingredient rather than the number of dose units as drugs are often presented in different formulations containing different amounts of active drug.

For example, furosemide tablets are available as 20 mg, 40 mg and 500 mg tablet strengths. Prescribing one tablet without describing the strength of the tablet will not specify the dose of furosemide the prescriber intends the patient to take.

Liquid medicines are often presented in concentrations which enable a 5 ml dose to be taken. A prescription for amoxicillin syrup 5 ml three times day does not specify the dose of amoxicillin the patient requires.

Guidance on the way in which doses should be expressed in prescriptions is given in the BNF.

Unnecessary use of decimal points should be avoided.

A decimal point is essential to prescribe a dose of 1.5 mg. However, prescribing a dose of 3 mg by writing 3.0 mg introduces an unnecessary decimal point. 3.0 mg could be misinterpreted as 30 mg, resulting in a tenfold overdose.

If a dose of less than one gram is needed the dose should be written in milligrams rather than parts of a gram, e.g. 300 mg not 0.3 g.

Doses of less than a milligram should be written as micrograms, e.g. 100 micrograms not 0.1 mg.

Where it is necessary to use a decimal point it should always be preceded by a zero. If the decimal point is not preceded by a zero it may be overlooked resulting in a tenfold overdose.

For example, the dose of alfacalcidol for hypocalcaemia is usually **0.**25–1 microgram daily. One Alpha® injection contains 1 microgram alfacalcidol in **0.**5 ml.

For some medicines which contain fixed combinations of drugs, or where the strength of the drug is described in the drug name, it is acceptable to specify the dose in terms of the number of dose units the patient should take.

For example, preparations of levodopa and carbidopa used in the treatment of Parkinson's disease contain these two drugs in a range of combinations so that symptom control can be titrated to the patient's needs.

Co-caryldopa 25/100 contains 25 mg carbidopa and 100 mg levodopa. It will be prescribed as co-caryldopa 25/100, one tablet to be taken three times a day. The amount of drug to be taken is specified in the drug name.

Table 14.2 lists other products which are commonly prescribed as the number of dose units.

The BNF suggests that the words micrograms and nanograms should not be abbreviated. However, the abbreviation 'mcg' is often used in electronic prescribing systems.

Table 14.2 Other products which are commonly prescribed as the number of dose units

Drug name	Ingredients	Typical dose
Co-dydramol	10 mg dihydrocodeine/500 mg paracetamol	1–2 tablets every six hours if required for pain
Co-tenidone	50 mg atenolol/12.5 mg chlorthalidone	1 tablet in the morning
Co-amilofruse 2.5/20	2.5 mg amiloride/20 mg furosemide	1 tablet in the morning
Co-amilofruse 5/50	5 mg amiloride/40 mg furosemide	1 tablet in the morning
Combivir®	300 mg zidovudine/150 mg lamivudine	1 tablet three times a day (adults)
Co-amoxiclav 375	125 mg clavulanic acid/250 mg amoxicillin	1 tablet three times a day
Co-amoxiclav 625	125 mg clavulanic acid/500 mg amoxicillin	1 tablets three times a day

Table 14.3 Morphine can be prescribed in a wide range of doses

Method of administration	Dose
Intravenous injection to a child	100–200 micrograms/kg (= 1–2 mg for a 10 kg child)
Subcutaneous injection to an adult	5–10 mg
Orally as MST Continus tablets in adults with chronic pain	5–200 mg (or more) every 12 hours
Subcutaneously as an infusion in palliative care	15–600 mg (or more) over 24 hours

For most drugs, confusion between milligrams and micrograms or micrograms and nanograms is unlikely to result in a dosing error as the difference in magnitude between these units is 1000. If a dose of 100 mcg was confused with 100 mg the patient would need to be given 1000 tablets to make up the dose, which will invariably be identified before the patient receives the dose.

Confusion with decimal point placement resulting in tenfold overdoses is more hazardous as it is less likely to be identified before a potentially harmful dose is administered to a patient. Tenfold overdoses are potential risks when calculating dilutions and infusion rates for injectable medicines and doses for children, especially for drugs with wide dose ranges, e.g. morphine (see Table 14.3).

Insulin and heparin are both high-risk drugs where adverse drug events can result in catastrophic patient harm. Serious patient harm has resulted from tenfold overdoses where the word 'units' or 'international units' have been abbreviated in the prescription (Table 14.4). For example, a prescription written as 4 u may be read as 40, and 4 iu may be read as 41 u. Similarly, with heparins 5000 u may be read as 50 000.

The word units must not be abbreviated in prescriptions.

Unusual frequencies

Most medicines are taken once a day or more frequently. For some indications medicines are prescribed less often than once a day, for example, weekly alendronate and risedronate for the treatment of postmenopausal osteoporosis, weekly oral methotrexate for the treatment of rheumatoid arthritis or psoriasis, and alternate day cotrimoxazole for prophylaxis of

Table 14.4 Poorly written abbreviations may result in tenfold overdoses

Dose ⟨7u⟩	7u looks like 70
Dose ⟨7 o⟩	Looks like 70 (the prescriber has used the symbol for a blood unit)
Dose ⟨7 iu⟩	7 iu looks like 71 u
Dose ⟨7 units⟩	Could be interpreted as mls
Dose ⟨7 units⟩	The word units should be written in full ideally with a space between the number and the word 'units'

Table 14.5 Variability of dosing schedules for drugs with unusual frequencies

Alendronate 10 mg daily	Alendonate 70 mg weekly
Risedronate 5 mg daily	Risedronate 35 mg weekly
Cotrimoxazole 960 mg twice daily	Cotrimoxazole 960 mg three times a week
Goserelin 3.6 mg every 28 days	Goserelin 10.8 mg every 12 weeks
Pentamidine nebulised 600 mg daily	Pentamidine nebulised 300 mg once a month

Pneumocystis carinii infections. These drugs can also be prescribed daily for different indications, introducing the risk of inadvertent daily dosing where weekly dosing is intended. Harmful errors have occurred where weekly dosing schedules have been misinterpreted as daily schedules.

A patient who should have been taking 17.5 mg methotrexate weekly (7×2.5 mg tablets) requested a change to her dosing regimen to try to reduce this tablet burden. The GP planned to prescribe her some 10 mg methotrexate tablets to take weekly along with 3×2.5 mg tablets to maintain her usual dose but accidentally prescribed 10 mg daily. Because the prescribing system did not have any built-in warning systems, the error was not noticed, nor was it noticed by the community pharmacist when the daily dose was dispensed. Within a week the patient had become unwell and she subsequently died of a gastrointestinal haemorrhage, pancytopaenia and methotrexate toxicity (Cambridgeshire Health Authority 2000).

Table 14.5 shows how dosing schedules for drugs can vary.

Electronic prescribing systems can be programmed to ensure that drugs are prescribed at the correct frequency. However, errors can occur with electronic prescribing systems without decision support and where prescriptions are handwritten where there is nothing to alert the prescriber that a potentially harmful prescribing error has occurred. If prescribers are unaware of the usual dose and frequency of a drug it is easy to assume that the dose is taken once daily and prescribe accordingly.

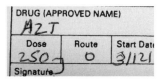

Figure 14.3 Abbreviated drug names may lead to incorrect assumptions

On hospital drug charts which are designed to support frequent drug dosing, doses not due must be crossed out to clearly indicate that they are not to be given.

Abbreviations and approved names

The BNF suggests that 'the names of drugs and preparations should be written clearly and not abbreviated, using approved titles only' (BNF 2008).

The use of abbreviated drug names can result in wrong drug errors, especially if the abbreviation used is not universally recognised and is liable to be misinterpreted.

The most well known example of a problematic drug name abbreviation is the abbreviation 'AZT' (see Figure 14.3). Azidothymidine is the chemical name of the drug zidovudine, an antiretroviral, and during clinical trials it was given the abbreviated name AZT. Although this abbreviation is still widely used and well recognised by people who regularly prescribe the drug it has been misinterpreted in other situations as an abbreviation for other drug names which include the letters A, Z and T, e.g. azathioprine (an immunosuppressant), azithromycin and aztreonam (both antibiotics). Abbreviated drug names should not be used without agreement and standardisation within a particular setting, ensuring everyone is aware of the meaning of the abbreviation, to avoid the risk of misinterpretation and drug error.

Using abbreviated drug names is actively discouraged and pharmacists and nurses should not be put into a position where they have to interpret a prescriber's shorthand before they dispense or administer a medicine. Do not abbreviate drug names.

The use of approved (generic) names is encouraged other than in situations where different brands of the same drug are not interchangeable because of differences in their pharmacokinetic profiles.

The BNF states within drug monographs where prescribing by brand name is preferred. For example, for longer-acting formulations of diltiazem, the BNF states:

> Different versions of modified-release preparations may not have the same clinical effect. To avoid confusion between these different formulations of diltiazem, prescribers should specify the brand to be dispensed (BNF 2008).

Also, there are situations where it is preferable to specify the brand name of a drug where there are several formulations of that drug available. Morphine sulphate and oxycodone are available in both immediate-release and modified-release formulations. Modified-release formulations are usually administered twice daily and immediate-release formulations are administered more frequently for an immediate effect. There is often confusion between the different formulations of these two drugs, resulting in the wrong formulation being prescribed or administered. Specifying the brand name, e.g. MSTContinus® or Sevredol®, Oxynorm® or Oxycontin®, in addition to the approved name when prescribing these preparations may reduce the risk of confusion, ensuring patients receive the correct medicine.

Table 14.6 Essential requirements for controlled drug prescriptions

	What you want the patient to have	Information the prescription must include
Drug name	Morphine sulphate (MST Continus®)	Morphine sulphate (MST Continus®)
Form		**Modified release tablets**
Strength		**30 mg tablets**
Dose and frequency	30 mg twice a day	30 mg twice a day
Quantity to be supplied	For two weeks	**28 tablets**
		Twenty-eight tablets
Signature	*A Prescriber*	*A Prescriber*
Date	A Date	A Date

The Medicines and Healthcare products Regulatory Agency have warned practitioners to be aware of the risk of confusion between two formulations of tacrolimus, Advagraf® and Prograf®, used as an immunosuppressant in organ transplantation. The two products are not interchangeable and errors resulting in patients taking the wrong formulation have led to serious adverse reactions including biopsy-confirmed acute rejection of transplanted organs. Again the risks of confusion may be reduced if the brand name is used to prescribe this critical drug (MHRA 2008).

Prescribing controlled drugs

Prescribing controlled drugs is something that even the most highly qualified prescribers sometimes find difficult. Although prescription of controlled drugs differs to the prescription of other drugs and some information included in the prescription is required by law, it is not difficult.

All well-written prescriptions must include the drug name, the dose, the frequency, the prescriber's signature and the date of prescription, and this includes controlled drugs.

The only additional information a controlled drug prescription must include is the *form and strength* of the drug, e.g. capsules, ampoules, liquid, patches, modified-release tablets and the *quantity* of that dosage form to be supplied, written in words and figures (see Table 14.6).

The quantity must refer to the form of the drug being given (tablets or mls in the examples above) and not to the number of milligrams of drug being supplied.

Electronic prescribing systems in primary care will generate prescriptions for controlled drugs which comply with the legal requirements for controlled drug prescriptions. However, when handwriting prescriptions, prescribers are responsible for supplying the additional information required. Pharmacists are not allowed to dispense a controlled drug unless all the required information is given on the prescription. Incomplete or illegal prescriptions can cause inconvenience to patients who will be unable to be supplied with their medicines.

In conclusion, to minimise the risk of patient harm, prescribers not only have responsibility for selecting the most appropriate course of treatment for patients under their care; they also have the responsibility of ensuring that their intentions are communicated to other practitioners in a clear and unambiguous way.

References

British National Formulary (2008). *Guidance on prescribing*. London: BMJ Group and RPS Publishing.

Cambridgeshire Health Authority (2000). Methotrexate toxicity. An inquiry into the death of a Cambridgeshire patient in April 2000. http://www.blacktriangle.org/methotrexate-toxicity.pdf (accessed 8 April 2009).

Charatan, F. (1999). Family compensated for death after illegible prescription. *BMJ* 319: 1456.

Dean, B., Barber, N., Schachter, M. (2000). What is a prescribing error? *Qual Health Care 9*: 232–237.

Institute for Safe Medication Practices (2005). *ISMP's List of Confused Drug Names*. http://www.ismp.org/tools/confuseddrugnames.pdf (accessed 8 April 2009).

Medicines and Healthcare products Regulatory Agency (2008). Prograf and Advagraf (tacrolimus): serious medication errors. *Drug Safety Update 2*(5).

National Patient Safety Agency (2007). *Safety in Doses: Medication Safety Incidents in the NHS*. London: NPSA.

Index